AF625040

Radiation Disaster Medicine

Koichi Tanigawa • Rethy Kieth Chhem
Editors

Radiation Disaster Medicine

Perspective from the Fukushima Nuclear Accident

Springer

Editors
Koichi Tanigawa
Department of Emergency and Critical Care Medicine
Hiroshima University
Hiroshima
Japan

Rethy Kieth Chhem
Division of Human Health
International Atomic Energy Agency
Vienna
Austria

ISBN 978-3-319-02215-4 ISBN 978-3-319-02216-1 (eBook)
DOI 10.1007/978-3-319-02216-1
Springer Heidelberg Dordrecht London New York

Library of Congress Control Number: 2013955234

© Springer International Publishing Switzerland 2014
This work is subject to copyright. All rights are reserved by the Publisher, whether the whole or part of the material is concerned, specifically the rights of translation, reprinting, reuse of illustrations, recitation, broadcasting, reproduction on microfilms or in any other physical way, and transmission or information storage and retrieval, electronic adaptation, computer software, or by similar or dissimilar methodology now known or hereafter developed. Exempted from this legal reservation are brief excerpts in connection with reviews or scholarly analysis or material supplied specifically for the purpose of being entered and executed on a computer system, for exclusive use by the purchaser of the work. Duplication of this publication or parts thereof is permitted only under the provisions of the Copyright Law of the Publisher's location, in its current version, and permission for use must always be obtained from Springer. Permissions for use may be obtained through RightsLink at the Copyright Clearance Center. Violations are liable to prosecution under the respective Copyright Law.
The use of general descriptive names, registered names, trademarks, service marks, etc. in this publication does not imply, even in the absence of a specific statement, that such names are exempt from the relevant protective laws and regulations and therefore free for general use.
While the advice and information in this book are believed to be true and accurate at the date of publication, neither the authors nor the editors nor the publisher can accept any legal responsibility for any errors or omissions that may be made. The publisher makes no warranty, express or implied, with respect to the material contained herein.

Disclaimer: The views and opinions expressed in this book are solely that of the editors and authors and are not representative of the views and opinions of the International Atomic Energy Agency, Hiroshima University, or any other institutions involved. This book is intended for educational and informational purposes only and should not be construed as medical advice. Information in this book is not a substitute for professional diagnosis or treatment. Please consult your physician before beginning any course of action based on the topics covered in this book.

Printed on acid-free paper

Springer is part of Springer Science+Business Media (www.springer.com)

Foreword

“Radiation emergency medicine,” in the modern sense of the word, began in Japan with the reception, triage, and overall medical management of three victims from the Tokai-mura criticality accident in 1999. Following this event, Japan’s radiation emergency medical preparedness and response system had been drastically restructured. It was the system unique to Japan, coincident with its Emergency Medical Services (EMS) system, and comprised the echelon of facilities and care from primary to tertiary. At the same time, a well-structured training program has been actively carried out since 2001, targeting medical, EMS personnel, local officials, and others for the first response to radiological emergencies. The assumed worst scenario was that of the Three Mile Island Nuclear Power Plant accident. One drawback was that the system as well as training and even the drills were in effect only in localities where the nuclear facility was located. Thus, the system could have been termed that of “radiation emergency medicine.”

Then the Fukushima Daiichi Nuclear Power Plant accident occurred, combined with the earthquake and subsequent tsunami. Admittedly, it caused great confusion in the immediate medical response because it was far beyond what had been expected and planned. However, the medico-social responses in Fukushima were nothing really new but something revisited. Things similar to what has been done in Fukushima in terms of disaster medical response were first practiced in the Chernobyl disaster in the former Soviet Union in 1986 and thereafter and then in the 1987 Goiania accident in Brazil. Namely, there were various radioprotective measures for the public and the environment on an extremely large scale where some medical involvement was inevitably required: sheltering, evacuation, stable iodide administration, radiation survey, decontamination, food and water restriction, relocation, etc.

Thus, the medical management of the various aspects of a nuclear disaster in its acute stage such as practiced in these events can be defined as “radiation disaster medicine.”

It is not just “radiation emergency medicine” but encompasses the medical involvement in those activities unique to nuclear disaster in addition to common issues with other disasters. Theoretically it can be considered as the on-scene application of knowledge and skills, among others, in emergency medicine, disaster medicine, radiology, psychiatry, and public health. In actuality, however, we have not discussed or studied systematically this area of the comprehensive medico-social response to a combined natural and nuclear disaster.

From the Tokai-mura criticality accident experience, we learned that the human network established ahead of time was crucially important to better deal with the difficult situation since the human resources in this field were scant. Most authors of this book have known each other through this human network and are credible experts small in number.

There are a few textbooks or manuals on radiation emergency medicine; however, they are not always based on the actual experience, have not stood the test of time, and usually presuppose an intact medical system.

In a sense, this book is the first effort of its kind. This book is not just a textbook but contains the actual descriptions of what responders and others had to do or what they have found at various points in time and at various places during and after this unprecedented, most severe nuclear accident in history. A nuclear accident causes far greater sociopsychological effects than other disasters, and it is well known that equal emphasis should be placed on psychological and physical health care of the affected.

Physicians and medical personnel may be driven to play the key role in communicating with the public in the relevant and timely fashion to alleviate their anxiety and fear.

These two important aspects of the medical response to a nuclear disaster are well described in this book, and the chapters serve as a good reference. Readers can better understand what actually happens in a radiation disaster, particularly caused by a major nuclear power plant accident. Readers may also refer to this book as the "ABC" in radiation disaster medicine as they prepare for the worst nuclear disaster scenario. It is hoped that readers will find this a useful reference.

Tsurushi, Japan Kazuhiko Maekawa, M.D.

Preface

There are many books available on "Disaster Medicine," but to the best of our knowledge, there is currently no book available that addresses "Radiation Disaster Medicine." The idea for this book was born from a discussion between the two editors while attending the "International Academic Conference on Radiation Health Risk Management in Fukushima" held in Fukushima on 25–27 February 2013. The two of us have had frequent interactions with physicians from Fukushima Medical University, Hiroshima University, and Nagasaki University and a few other medical institutions in Japan. We have come to learn that during the initial phase of the accident, physicians and Japan Disaster Medical Assistance Teams provided medical relief in an extremely difficult environment; infrastructure including medical, transportation, water and electricity supplies, and communication systems were disrupted. We were impressed by the courage and sacrifice demonstrated by frontline responders. They provided emergency services in the midst of the combined disasters, putting their own life at risk, while the extent of radiation risk was still unknown.

The book *Radiation Disaster Medicine* provides an overarching conceptualization of the problem based on what we have learned from the Fukushima accident in particular which we believe will offer guidance for medical management during the acute phase of a radiation disaster. The concept includes understanding physicians' roles in radiation disasters (from micro and macro perspectives), imbuing lessons from past radiation disasters, and preparing for future radiation emergencies.

No clear definition of radiation disaster medicine has been articulated after the Chernobyl and Three Mile Island accidents. The radiation emergency medical system developed in Japan after the Three Mile Island and JCO accidents did not offer sufficient breadth or depth to manage the Fukushima accident, which was further complicated by the destruction caused by the combined natural disasters. Thus, many physicians were not sufficiently prepared to manage the Fukushima accident. This book offers an emphasis on medical and psychological readiness that is essential in mitigating any radiation disasters. Additionally, although no death from acute radiation syndrome was encountered in the Fukushima accident, there were unexpected casualties during evacuation and marked difficulties in medical management even though they were unrelated to radiation. An overarching purpose of this book is therefore to broaden the lens, examine the unique challenges that physicians face, and introduce readers to some key institutions in radiation disaster situations.

This book employs a comprehensive approach that includes medical basics and social considerations, covers all levels of emergency care (primary, secondary, tertiary), and clarifies common issues and specific considerations in radiation and other disasters. It is to be noted that this book should not be perceived as excluding disaster medical responses for other disasters but that it is especially focused on radiation disasters. *Radiation Disaster Medicine* is intended for health-care professionals, prehospital emergency care providers, and emergency personnel involved in responses.

Through this book, readers can better understand what happens in radiation disaster in order to provide appropriate management and care for those injured, evacuees, and residents. Knowledge of radiation disaster medicine is made up to date for health-care professionals in all fields, as well as recommended to be included into medical school curriculum for capacity building. Finally, an expected outcome would be minimization of confusion and misconceptions among emergency personnel and residents in the case of another radiation disaster.

Hiroshima, Japan — Koichi Tanigawa
Vienna, Austria — Rethy Kieth Chhem

Contents

1 **Physicians' Early Response to the Fukushima Daiichi Nuclear Power Plant Accident: Challenges and Lessons Learned** 1
Rethy Kieth Chhem

2 **General Considerations in Radiation Disaster Medicine** 15
Koichi Tanigawa

3 **Medical Perspective** 29
Koichi Tanigawa and Arifumi Hasegawa

4 **Disaster Behavioral Health: Psychological Effects of the Fukushima Nuclear Power Plant Accident** 79
Masaharu Maeda and Misari Oe

5 **Management Perspective: Structure of Radiation Emergency Response in Japan** 89
Takako Tominaga, Misao Hachiya, and Makoto Akashi

6 **Management Perspective: Structure of Radiation Emergency Response in International Organizations** 99
Azura Z. Aziz and Pisith Phlong

7 **Radiation Disaster Medicine Curriculum Revisited in a Post-Fukushima Context** 109
Rethy Kieth Chhem, Azura Z. Aziz, and Gregory K. Clancey

Index 121

Contributors

Koichi Tanigawa, M.D., Ph.D. Department of Emergency and Critical Care Medicine, Hiroshima University, Hiroshima, Japan

Rethy Kieth Chhem, M.D., Ph.D. (Edu), Ph.D. (His) Division of Human Health, International Atomic Energy Agency, Vienna, Austria

Fukushima Medical University, Fukushima, Japan

Hiroshima University, Hiroshima, Japan

Nagasaki University, Nagasaki, Japan

Institute of History, Philosophy and Ethics of Medicine, Ulm University, Ulm, Germany

Makoto Akashi, M.D., Ph.D. National Institute of Radiological Sciences (NIRS), Chiba, Japan

Azura Z. Aziz, B.Sc. (Hons) Division of Human Health, International Atomic Energy Agency, Vienna, Austria

Gregory K. Clancey, Ph.D. Asia Research Institute, National University of Singapore, Singapore, Singapore

Tembusu College, National University of Singapore, Singapore, Singapore

Misao Hachiya, Ph.D. Department of Radiation Emergency Medical Assistance Team (REMAT), National Institute of Radiological Sciences (NIRS), Chiba, Japan

Arifumi Hasegawa, M.D., Ph.D. Department of Emergency and Critical Care Medicine, Radiation Disaster Medical Center, Fukushima Medical University, Fukushima, Japan

Masaharu Maeda, M.D., Ph.D. Department of Neuropsychiatry, School of Medicine, Kurume University, Fukuoka, Japan

Department of Disaster Psychiatry, School of Medicine, Fukushima Medical University, Fukushima, Japan

Kazuhiko Maekawa, M.D., Ph.D. Tsuru-Tranomon Surgery & Rehabilitation Hospital, Tsurushi, Yamanashi, Japan

Misari Oe, M.D., Ph.D. Division of Health Services, Institute of Health and Sports Science, Kurume University, Fukuoka, Japan

Department of Neuropsychiatry, School of Medicine, Kurume University, Fukuoka, Japan

Pisith Phlong, M.A. (Anthropology) Division of Human Health, International Atomic Energy Agency, Vienna, Austria

Takako Tominaga, M.D., Ph.D. Department of Radiation Emergency Medical Assistance Team (REMAT), National Institute of Radiological Sciences (NIRS), Chiba, Japan

Abbreviations

ALARA	As Low as Reasonably Achievable
ARS	Acute Radiation Syndrome
APSTSN	Asia-Pacific Science, Technology and Society Network
CBRNE	Chemical, Biological, Radiological, Nuclear, and High-Yield Explosives
CDPC	Central Disaster Prevention Council
DMAT	Disaster Medical Assistance Team
DRD	Disaster-Related Death
ED	Emergency Department
ER	Emergency Room
FAO	Food and Agricultural Organization
FMU	Fukushima Medical University
GM	Geiger-Mueller
HS	Hematopoietic Syndrome
IAEA	International Atomic Energy Agency
ICRP	International Commission on Radiological Protection
IEC	Incident and Emergency Centre
IEComm	Operations Manual for Incident and Emergency Communication
ILO	International Labour Organization
INES	International Nuclear Event Scale
IO	International Organizations
JAAM	Japan Association for Acute Medicine
JFA	Japan Football Association
JMAT	Japan Medical Association
JPLAN	Joint Radiation Emergency Management Plan of the International Organizations
JSDF	Japan Self-Defense Force
LET	Linear Energy Transfer
LOC	Level of Consciousness
LRI	Local Radiation Injury
MCE	Mass Casualty Events
NAHU	Division of Human Health
NEA	Nuclear Energy Agency
NIRS	National Institute of Radiological Sciences

NPP	Nuclear Power Plant
NRA	Nuclear Regulation Authority
NSC	Nuclear Safety Commission
OCHA	The Office for the Coordination of Humanitarian Affairs
OFC	Off-site Center
PB	Persian Blue
PNC	Power Reactor and Nuclear Fuel Development Corporation
PPE	Personal Protective Equipment
PTSD	Post-traumatic Stress Disorder
RANET	Response and Assistance Network
REA	Radiation Emergency Area
REMAT	Radiation Emergency Medical Assistance Team
SPEEDI	System for Prediction of Environmental Emergency Dose Information
START	Simple Triage and Rapid Treatment
STS	Science and Technology Studies
TEPCO	Tokyo Electric Power Co.
TMI	Three Mile Island
UNEP	United Nations Environment Program
UNSCEAR	United Nations Scientific Committee on the Effects of Atomic Radiation
UPZ	Urgent Protective Action Planning Zone
WHO	World Health Organization
WMO	World Meteorological Organization

Physicians' Early Response to the Fukushima Daiichi Nuclear Power Plant Accident: Challenges and Lessons Learned

1

Rethy Kieth Chhem

Contents

1.1 Introduction 2
1.2 Physician as Expert 4
1.2.1 Experts in Radiation Disaster Medicine 4
1.2.2 Experts in Other Medical Fields 5
1.3 Physicians as Professionals 9
1.4 Physicians as Communicators 10
Conclusions 11
References 11

Abstract

Various roles of physicians in the early responses to the Fukushima Daiichi nuclear power plant accident were described and reviewed according to the competency-based framework of CanMEDS. It was found that most physicians from various medical specialties including radiation disaster medicine were unprepared to deal with a combination of disasters (earthquake and tsunami) compounded by a technological disaster due to the Fukushima Daiichi nuclear power

R.K. Chhem, M.D., Ph.D. (Edu), Ph.D. (His)
Division of Human Health, International Atomic Energy Agency, Wagramerstrasse 5, 200, Vienna A-1400, Austria

Fukushima Medical University, Fukushima, Japan

Hiroshima University, Hiroshima, Japan

Nagasaki University, Nagasaki, Japan

Institute of History, Philosophy and Ethics of Medicine, Ulm University, Ulm, Germany
e-mail: r.chhem@iaea.org

K. Tanigawa, R.K. Chhem (eds.), *Radiation Disaster Medicine*,
DOI 10.1007/978-3-319-02216-1_1, © Springer International Publishing Switzerland 2014

plant meltdown. Challenges and lessons learned in the wake of the Fukushima accident were also examined, whereby the weakest spot that has been identified by physicians on the front line is the ability to communicate effectively with various publics about the risk of radiation on human health.

1.1 Introduction

The purpose of this chapter is to describe various roles of physicians in the early responses to the Fukushima accident. This review is based on the analysis of written sources from the medical literature, abstracts from various scientific conferences on the Fukushima accident and its health consequences, and testimonies from physicians who have been involved in the early medical response to the accident. The results of this review may point to some patterns of the medical response to a major nuclear accident and consequently identify educational gaps that need to be addressed by reforming some aspects of the medical curriculum for physicians, as lack of proper knowledge in radiation among physicians led to some inappropriate interventions observed in many situations. The description of the roles of physicians is done according to the competency-based framework of CanMEDS (Table 1.1). I acknowledge the limitations of such an approach because the medical educational model in Japanese culture does not necessarily follow the pattern of Canadian physician training.

In addition to the generic principles of CanMEDS, the requirements of nuclear medicine physician training may be helpful because those specialists deal with radioactive sources that represent the main concern for health in case of a nuclear accident (Royal College of Physicians and Surgeons of Canada [RCPSC] 2009). Of all the seven competencies established for nuclear medicine physicians, communication skills seem to be the weakest spot identified among physicians working on the front line (Table 1.2). The key challenge faced by physicians in the wake of the Fukushima disaster is the ability to communicate effectively with various publics about the risk of radiation on human health. This key competence is an integral part of the Canadian nuclear medicine physician training. Public information about radiation effects is the responsibility of those medical specialists.

In order to understand the reality of the local conditions faced by physicians during the emergency phase of the medical response, I will use the anecdotal example of Iwaki Kyoritsu Hospital (Koyama et al. 2011) as a case in point to describe the crisis situation:

- Shortage of staff: Staff below the age of 40 were instructed to evacuate the city.
- Pharmacies in town were closed.
- Short supply of water; therefore, no surgical procedures were possible.
- Short supply of medicines.
- Hemodialysis services interrupted.
- Emergency calls not attended as fire department was overwhelmed by urgent tasks.
- Widespread rumors of contamination of the city.

Other related issues that arose in the wake of the Fukushima accident are (Gonzalez et al. 2013):

Table 1.1 The CanMEDS physician competency framework (Frank (ed) 2005)

Physician competencies	Description
Medical expert	"Physicians possess a defined body of knowledge, clinical skills, procedural skills and professional attitudes, which are directed to effective patient-centered care. They apply these competencies to collect and interpret information, make appropriate clinical decisions, and carry out diagnostic and therapeutic interventions"
Collaborator	"Physicians work in partnership with others who are appropriately involved in the care of individuals or specific groups of patients"
Communicator	"Physicians enable patient-centered therapeutic communication through shared decision-making and effective dynamic interactions with patients, families, caregivers, other professionals, and important other individuals. The competencies of this Role are essential for establishing rapport and trust, formulating a diagnosis, delivering information, striving for mutual understanding, and facilitating a shared plan of care"
Professional	"The Professional Role is guided by codes of ethics and a commitment to clinical competence, the embracing of appropriate attitudes and behaviors, integrity, altruism, personal well-being, and to the promotion of the public good within their domain. These commitments form the basis of a social contract between a physician and society. Society, in return, grants physicians the privilege of profession-led regulation with the understanding that they are accountable to those served"
Scholar	"Physicians engage in a lifelong pursuit of mastering their domain of expertise. As learners, they recognize the need to be continually learning and model this for others. Through their scholarly activities, they contribute to the creation, dissemination, application and translation of medical knowledge"
Health advocate	"Physicians recognize their duty and ability to improve the overall health of their patients and the society they serve. Doctors identify advocacy activities as important for the individual patient, for populations of patients and for communities. … Communities and societies need physicians' special expertise to identify and collaboratively address broad health issues and the determinants of health. At this level, health advocacy involves efforts to change specific practices or policies on behalf of those served. Framed in this multi-level way, health advocacy is an essential and fundamental component of health promotion. Health advocacy is appropriately expressed both by individual and collective actions of physicians in influencing public health and policy"
Manager	"Physicians interact with their work environment as individuals, as members of teams or groups, and as participants in the health system locally, regionally or nationally. The balance in the emphasis among these three levels varies depending on the nature of the specialty, but all specialties have explicitly identified management responsibilities as a core requirement for the practice of medicine in their discipline"

- Health professionals involved in emergency medicine did not have adequate basic understanding of radiation and radioactive elements.
- The core curriculum in medical schools was not suitable for radiological science training.
- Risk communication and education was insufficient.
- Ineffective medical preparedness, including drills and exercise.

Table 1.2 The CanMEDS training objectives for nuclear medicine residency program (RCPSC 2009)

Physician competency	Description
Communication	"Interact with the public, local advisory personnel and regulatory agencies to address procedural issues Present information to the public or media about a medical, radiation safety or regulatory issue, when appropriate Demonstrate the ability to provide sophisticated information about radiation safety, relative risk, or applicable regulations, at a knowledge or education-appropriate level in order to promote understanding of the issues and the discipline Communicate with appropriate local or national bodies, when necessary, to deal with issues as they arise"

In addition, lessons learned from the accident are as follows (Gonzalez et al. 2013):

- Health professionals should have at least a fundamental understanding of radioactivity and radiation and of their potential health effects.
- Physicians, nurses, radiation technologists, and first medical responders should have a basic understanding of radiation because any or all of these health professionals might be called upon to respond to the front line of a radiological emergency.

Within those circumstances and against all odds, physicians decided to evacuate selected patients, based on their medical conditions, by themselves. The team in charge of evacuation of patients from the hospital was made exclusively of physicians who even drove the ambulance themselves. This example of organized evacuation could not be conducted without an effective leadership displayed by physicians at this particular hospital.

Indeed one cannot generalize the pattern of medical response of physicians to the Fukushima accident from this single anecdotal case, but certainly one can measure the mismatch between the need and the resources in an overall situation of uncertainty.

1.2 Physician as Expert

According to CanMEDS (RCPSC 2005), the experts are physicians who:

> Possess a defined body of knowledge, clinical skills, procedural skills and professional attitudes, which are directed to effective patient-centered care. They apply these competencies to collect and interpret information, make appropriate clinical decisions, and carry out diagnostic and therapeutic interventions.

1.2.1 Experts in Radiation Disaster Medicine

The role of radiation disaster medicine experts is the subject of study of this book and will be addressed in specific chapters. The majority of those experts were involved in the clinical management of patients that were exposed to radiation. The scale and scope were overwhelming for a limited number of radiation specialists from the National Institute of Radiological Sciences (NIRS) and Hiroshima University and Nagasaki University hospitals. Beyond the clinical management of trauma patients (caused by tsunami and the earthquake) and patients who may have been exposed to radiation, a few senior radiation experts act as advisor to prefectural and central governments. Others serve as senior academic officers to assist University presidents to design proper academic responses based on the needs that were identified in the wake of the accident.

1.2.2 Experts in Other Medical Fields

Non-radiation medical specialist participation in the management of natural disasters like earthquake and tsunami is essential. Almost the entire spectrum of medical specialists was needed as well to assist in the management of the combined natural disaster and technological accident. Without being exhaustive, the review below demonstrates the numerous roles of physicians in the response to the Fukushima accident.

1.2.2.1 Radiologists, Nuclear Medicine Physicians, and Radio-Oncologists

Physicians specializing in radiology, nuclear medicine, and radio-oncology have been trained in the safe and effective use of radiation for medical diagnosis and treatment. They are most suitably equipped with knowledge and skills to address issues related to the consequences of radiation on human health – although they are not necessarily experts in radiation disaster medicine – and should therefore ideally constitute the team of emergency response medical experts in a radiation disaster. However, from a review of the literature in English, few of these specialists have been involved in the medical response to nuclear accidents in Chernobyl or Fukushima. Kereiakes et al. (1986) highlight the "very important role" of nuclear medicine specialists, but there is no indication of actual involvement of these specialists, just the likelihood and potential of their contribution to the Chernobyl medical response.

I recognize that, because of the language barrier, I have no access to Japanese publications about this important topic. From our literature search, only one article was published by a Japanese radiologist from Iwate Medical University for whom the response to the Fukushima accident was to act on patients who presented at his hospital (Ehara 2011). According to the information drawn from this limited number of publications, the role of "radiology professionals" in addressing nuclear accidents is recognized (American College of Radiology [ACR] 2006). The ACR document on disaster preparedness provides a clear body of theoretical knowledge on the medical response to a radiation accident and identifies those specialists as "sources of accurate information for patients, the public, and the medical community" (ACR 2006, p. 3). However, despite this declaration, the single most important issue of radiation, that is risk communication to the publics, is not addressed in the document. A review paper "Medical Response to a Major Radiologic Emergency" published by Radiology (Wolbarst et al. 2010) calls for the same contribution from "radiology specialists" to become advisors to policy makers or science communicators for the media. The review recognizes the need for an effective communication strategy. Yet again, radiologists are not taught on what and how to tell the publics when they have been asked whether it is safe or not to live in a certain area nearby the accident site.

In order for radiology specialists to be effective in medical responses to radiation disasters, training for public communication is necessary. At the standpoint of risk communication, radiology specialists are primarily taught to communicate with patients in the context of radiation in diagnostics and medical treatment on a one-to-one basis (Ohno 2010; Staudenherz and Sinzinger 2012). Currently, public communication within the context of scientific uncertainty and public mistrust is also increasingly emphasized in radiation disaster medicine that does not only teach radiology specialists to provide the publics with information about radiation exposure (Staudenherz and Sinzinger 2012).

1.2.2.2 Emergency Physicians

Emergency medicine covers diverse areas from various diseases requiring emergency treatment in the emergency department (ED) to pre-hospital care. In Japan, emergency specialty has been developed as a discipline called "Acute Medicine," which features continuity of trauma and critical care from pre-hospital, ED, and intensive care unit (Safar 1974; Japanese Association for Acute Medicine 2007). Although the scope of practice of emergency specialties may vary from country to country, physicians in the emergency arena are frequently involved with disaster preparedness and countermeasures.

In the Great East Japan earthquake, approximately 24,000 medical personnel were involved in medical activities in the Tohoku region during the first 2 months after the earthquake (see Chap. 3) (Ministry of Health, Labor, and Welfare 2011). However, only a small number of emergency physicians headed for Fukushima soon after the accident because concerns over radiation existed, and information on radiation was not properly shared. In addition, most of them had not been properly trained for radiation disasters.

Although only a few were available, emergency physicians who were trained in disaster medicine as well as radiation emergency were at the core of the subsequent medical responses dealing with the most difficult situation in the Fukushima accident (Tanigawa et al. 2011a, b).

The roles of emergency physicians in radiation disaster are clear: planning for pre-hospital and hospital responses, medical activities on the scene and at hospitals, and coordination in responses as medical advisors at the operation center, hospitals, and disaster headquarters. In order to achieve these tasks effectively, emergency physicians should understand the nature of radiation, and the impacts of radiation disaster on individuals and societies.

1.2.2.3 Family and Community Physicians

The current primary care system in Japan is not as developed as it should be as most patients accede to health care either through the hospitals or specialist consultation. As a result, hospital facilities were quickly overwhelmed in the wake of the disasters by an influx of patients who may not have needed urgent or specialized care in secondary or tertiary cares centers (Starkey and Maeda 2011). The emergency situation caused by both the disasters and evacuation was compounded by the rush of many patients to health-care centers (clinics or small-sized hospitals) or in evacuation shelters, where their medical records were not available, especially the electronic patient records that were not accessible because of the shutoff of electricity supply. In most situations, family physicians relied only on their clinical skills to diagnose and treat patients (Ishii 2013, p. 92). Laboratory or X-ray tests were also not available because of the cutoff of electricity and water supplies. The main casualties seen were drowning followed by trauma caused by building and house collapses (Ishii 2013, p. 94). The biggest challenge was the inadequacy of the scale of medical needs in evacuation centers and the availability of physicians rotating among evacuation centers (Ishii 2013, pp. 94–95).

1.2.2.4 Geriatricians

It is well known that elderly patients are more vulnerable to evacuation and relocation. Excess of mortality among relocated elderly after the Fukushima accident was documented (Yasumura et al. 2013). Pneumonia was the main cause of mortality. During the emergency phase, the causes of mortality during and after evacuation were hypothermia, dehydration, and deterioration of underlying medical conditions (Tanigawa et al. 2012). Most geriatric patients are affected by one or more chronic diseases that require long-term and continuous medications. One of the other main challenges faced by geriatricians in the wake of the Fukushima accident was to secure a stable supply of essential drugs for their elderly patients especially in shelters for evacuees. Because of the breakdown of the telephone network, communication was done through the use of the Internet (e-mail, Skype, or Twitter). For example, geriatricians were able to notify displaced patients through Twitter and advise them on where to get their medications. Through Tweets or "re-Tweet" communication system, dissemination of relevant information was relatively easy to achieve which enabled geriatricians to overcome the breakdown of the medication supply system much more effectively (Tamura and Fukuda 2011). Another major clinical situation that compounds the difficulties in providing services for the elderly patients is the need for much more extensive psychological support (Furukawa and Arai 2011). This topic will be addressed elsewhere in this chapter.

1.2.2.5 Hematologists and Transfusion Medicine Physicians

Hematologists and transfusion medicine physicians play specific roles in the wake of disasters. Many traumatic patients will need blood transfusion. In disaster situations, maintaining a regular and smooth blood supply, despite the disruption of basic means of transportation, is the top priority for experts in transfusion medicine. Red blood cells and frozen plasma are stocked in the hospital. The Fukushima Medical University was well equipped to collect platelets and whole blood for autologous patients. Because one-way HLA match is higher in Japanese than other populations, irradiation of allogeneic blood is common (Nollet 2013). Initially, there was provision made by the Japan Society for Hematopoietic Cells

Transplantation to create 107 transplant teams to eventually collect and store stem cells from peripheral blood for TEPCO workers. However, the Nuclear Safety Commission suggested that there was no such need for the workers whose treatment may indicate this kind of treatment (Tanimoto et al. 2011).

1.2.2.6 Orthopedic Surgeons and Anesthetists

Orthopedic surgeons are well trained in the management of traumatic injuries from building and house collapses during earthquakes, especially in Japan. The first priority is to save life, i.e., treating patients with internal bleeding and injuries. Life-saving surgical treatments are provided by trauma surgeons or emergency surgeons. Once stabilized and when necessary, the patient is referred to the orthopedic surgeons for orthopedic trauma like fractures and dislocations (Iwamoto 2012). The severity of the fractures and the experience of the surgical team, operating in extreme conditions of disasters, condition the outcome of the limb salvage surgical procedures. Indeed, no surgical procedures could be performed without the assistance of a competent anesthetic team.

1.2.2.7 Pulmonary Specialists

Besides the challenges of treating pneumonia in elderly patients living in shelters, their major concern consisted of securing the supply of inhaled corticosteroids. Pulmonary specialists worked closely with the Japanese authorities to reestablish an effective drug supply system in order to save asthma patients' lives in case of severe respiratory crises. Hence, the Japanese government established new policies to exceptionally allow pharmacists to deliver antiasthmatic drugs without any need for a physician's prescription (Fukuhara et al. 2013, p. 176).

1.2.2.8 Nephrologists

Nephrologists play two main roles in the case of major disasters. Firstly they participate in the management of patients with crush syndrome complicated by acute renal failure. Secondly, because routine hemodialysis service is disrupted in a disaster situation, the role of nephrologists is to restore dialysis facilities (Fukagawa et al. 2013). Therefore 600 dialysis patients from Iwaki were transferred to Niigata, 200 km away, where nephrologists were well experienced in practicing hemodialysis in the wake of two previous earthquakes that occurred there in 2004 and 2007. Because most patients had been evacuated in a hurry, there were no medical records available to guide urgent hemodialysis, so nephrologists made their therapeutic decisions on the basis of medical history and mere clinical examination of the patients (Kazama and Narita 2011).

1.2.2.9 Pediatricians

Like elderly patients, children are also extremely vulnerable in the wake of a major disaster. In Koriyama City, two hospitals were heavily damaged by the earthquake. Sick children had to be evacuated via the emergency stairway. Critically ill patients were evacuated to proper medical centers by private cars. Besides local patients, 5,000 evacuees were relocated in Koriyama City. Pediatricians played many roles:

doing rounds, providing emergency care, and supporting other doctors in secondary care hospitals. A major preoccupation of pediatricians was to prevent the development of posttraumatic stress disorders in children. Expertise from a few child psychiatrists and clinical psychologists was also sought to address that urgent issue (Kikuchi and Kikuchi 2012).

1.2.2.10 Psychiatrists

The roles of psychiatric specialists in the wake of a disaster are to provide mental health services to psychiatric patients and to give psychosocial support to the wider population (Takeda 2011). Their main issues of concern in the acute phase were the continuation of medication and treatment for current psychiatric patients and necessary drug supply, as well as the treatment of acute stress disorders. Fifty-seven volunteer mental health teams consisting of psychiatrists, nurses, psychologists, and/or social workers, who were equipped to be self-sufficient and self-supporting, were dispatched to refugee shelters in affected areas to address these concerns (Suzuki and Kim 2012). The teams also treated people who were recovering from the disaster through psycho-education, supportive counseling, and temporary medication for behavioral symptoms (Kim 2011).

1.2.2.11 Occupational Health Physicians (TEPCO Workers)

Occupational health physicians have specific expertise for protecting the lives and health of workers related to the workplace, notably in a complex disaster situation. Occupational health physicians were dispatched to a building at the Fukushima nuclear power plant for daily first aid services and periodic health checkups for TEPCO workers for iodine sensitivity, previous thyroid conditions (Wada et al. 2012), and radiation exposure (Mori et al. 2013). Volunteer physicians were based at the Fukushima nuclear power plant site to respond immediately to heat stroke and injuries and to refer severe cases to designated secondary or tertiary hospitals. Occupational health physicians also provided behavioral health examinations for TEPCO workers (Wada et al. 2012).

1.3 Physicians as Professionals

According to CanMEDS (RCPSC 2005), professionals are those who are:

> Guided by codes of ethics and a commitment to clinical competence, the embracing of appropriate attitudes and behaviors, integrity, altruism, personal well-being, and to the promotion of the public good within their domain. These commitments form the basis of a social contract between a physician and society. Society, in return, grants physicians the privilege of profession-led regulation with the understanding that they are accountable to those served.

Beyond clinical competence per se, the most striking question regarding physicians' professionalism according to CanMEDS is related to the physicians' respective attitudes vis-à-vis the Fukushima accident, i.e., if the accident poses an immediate threat both to the public and to the physicians themselves. In the wake of the Fukushima accident, the question for physicians was "To be in Fukushima, or not to be?" That was the question for some physicians practicing in the prefecture (Akabayashi 2012; Akabayashi et al. 2012). A survey conducted in late July 2012 by an association of Fukushima prefecture hospitals shows that hundreds of physicians and nurses have resigned. The number of physicians from Fukushima City dropped from 441 to 400, Minami-Soma from 28 to 15, Koriyama from 312 to 287, and Iwaki from 134 to 103 (The Yomiuri Shimbun 4 October 2011). In response to the decline in the numbers of physicians and nurses, the Fukushima prefectural government allocated extra funding for recruitment of extra staff to maintain adequate health-care services in the prefecture.

1.4 Physicians as Communicators

According to CanMEDS (RCPSC 2009):

> Physicians enable patient-centered therapeutic communication through shared decision-making and effective dynamic interactions with patients, families, caregivers, other professionals, and important other individuals. The competencies of this role are essential for establishing rapport and trust, formulating a diagnosis, delivering information, striving for mutual understanding, and facilitating a shared plan of care.

CanMEDS guidelines are clear in terms of providing physicians with communication skills that are unfortunately limited to addressing the needs of the patient himself/herself or his/her family. Unfortunately, the act of informing a large public about health issues, especially in the wake of a natural disaster compounded by a nuclear accident, is not part of any medical specialist training from the CanMEDS perspective. However, this key competence is an integral part of the Canadian nuclear medicine physician training. Public information about radiation effects is the responsibility of those medical specialists. The residency program stipulates clearly that a nuclear medicine physician must be able to (RCPSC 2009):

> Interact with the public, local advisory personnel and regulatory agencies to address procedural issues
>
> - Present information to the public or media about a medical, radiation safety or regulatory issue, when appropriate
> - Demonstrate the ability to provide sophisticated information about radiation safety, relative risk, or applicable regulations, at a knowledge or education-appropriate level in order to promote understanding of the issues and the discipline
> - Communicate with appropriate local or national bodies, when necessary, to deal with issues as they arise

As discussed earlier in this chapter, radiology specialists (radiologists, nuclear medicine physicians, radiation oncologists, as well as medical radiation physicists) constitute the ideal group to be trained in "nuclear science communications" with the task of informing various publics, in order to guide the respective publics towards an enlightened decision in the midst of a nuclear disaster. Medical radiation physicists are not physicians, but they work closely with health professionals and are trained in radiation dosimetry; thus, they are able to contribute to radiation disaster recovery efforts (Meghzifene and Nuesslin 2011). The assistance of professionals like these science communicators is essential to this endeavor. The expected outcome will be radiology specialists equipped with the skills and attitude necessary to communicate science and controversial technology to the public in an effective way. These specialists will take into consideration the uncertainty of scientific prediction and the inevitable mistrust of scientific and political authority post-disaster, especially when radiation is involved.

Conclusions

In this chapter, challenges faced during the early medical response to the Fukushima accident are identified and recognized. Lessons learned in the wake of the disaster serves as a foundation for academic and medical response, which will be elaborated upon in Chap. 8.

Acknowledgments The author would like to acknowledge Professor Koichi Tanigawa for his contribution of the emergency physician subsection, as well as ideas and guidance for this chapter. The author would also like to thank Ms. Azura Z. Aziz for her assistance in bibliographic research and editing.

References

Akabayashi A (2012) Must I stay? The obligations of physicians in proximity to the Fukushima nuclear power plant. Camb Q Healthc Ethics 21(3):392–395. doi:10.1017/S0963180112000126

Akabayashi A, Takimoto Y, Hayashi Y (2012) Physician obligation to provide care during disasters: should physicians have been required to go to Fukushima? J Med Ethics 38(11):697–698. doi:10.1136/medethics-2011-100216

American College of Radiology (2006) Disaster preparedness for radiology professionals: response to radiological terrorism. Retrieved from http://www.acr.org/~/media/ACR/Documents/PDF/Membership/Legal%20Business/Disaster%20Preparedness/Primer.pdf

Ehara S (2011) In a radiology department during the earthquake, tsunami, and the nuclear power plant accident. Am J Roentgenol 197:W549–W550. doi:10.2214/AJR.11.7004

Frank JR (ed) (2005) The CanMEDS 2005 physician competency framework: better standards, better physicians, better care. The Royal College of Physicians and Surgeons of Canada, Ottawa

Fukagawa M, Kim JI, Fujii H (2013) Another role for nephrologists in disaster medicine. Clin Exp Nephrol 12(2):153–154. doi:10.1007/s10157-013-0773-0

Fukuhara A, Sato S, Uematsu M, Misa K, Nikaido T, Inokoshi Y et al (2013) Impacts of the 3/11 disaster in Fukushima on asthma control. In: Fukushima: lives on the line – a compendium of reports from the 2011 Great East Japan earthquake and tsunami. Minpo, Fukushima, pp 176–177

Furukawa K, Arai H (2011) Earthquake in Japan. Lancet 377(9778):1652. doi:10.1016/S0140-6736(11)60671-5

Gonzalez AJ, Akashi M, Boice JD Jr et al (2013) Radiological protection issues arising during and after the Fukushima nuclear reactor accident. J Radiol Prot 33(3):497–571 (Epub ahead of print)

Ishii A (2013) People cannot live alone. In: Fukushima: lives on the line – a compendium of reports from the 2011 Great East Japan earthquake and tsunami. Minpo, Fukushima, pp 92–97

Iwamoto Y (2012) What should we do as orthopaedic surgeons in catastrophic disasters? J Orthop Sci 17(1):1–2. doi:10.1007/s00776-011-0195-3
Japanese Association for Acute Medicine (2007) Specialist system: emergency doctor. http://www.jaam.jp/html/senmoni/ideal.htm. Accessed 12 July 2013 (in Japanese)
Kazama JJ, Narita I (2011) Earthquake in Japan. Lancet 377(9778):1653. doi:10.1016/S0140-6736(11)60673-9
Kereiakes JG, Saenger EL, Thomas SR (1986) The reactor accident at Chernobyl: a nuclear medicine practitioner's perspective. Semin Nucl Med 16(3):224–230
Kikuchi S, Kikuchi T (2012) The medical association activity and paediatric care after the earthquake disaster in Fukushima. Keio J Med 61(1):23–27
Kim Y (2011) Great East Japan earthquake and early mental-health-care response. Psychiatry Clin Neurosci 65(6):539–548. doi:10.1111/j.1440-1819.2011.02270.x
Koyama A, Fuse A, Hagiwara J, Matsumoto G, Shiraishi S, Masuno T et al (2011) Medical relief activities, medical resourcing, and inpatient evacuation conducted by Nippon Medical School due to the Fukushima Daiichi Nuclear Power Plant accident following the Great East Japan Earthquake 2011. J Nippon Med Sch 78(6):393–396
Meghzifene A, Nuesslin F (2011) Do medical physicists have a role in case of a nuclear or radiological emergency? Phys Med 27(3):121. doi:10.1016/j.ejmp.2011.06.001
Ministry of Health, Labor and Welfare (2011) Report on damages and medical responses in 2011 off the Pacific coast of Tohoku Earthquake, Tohoku (in Japanese)
Mori K, Tateishi S, Hiraoka K, Kubo T, Okazaki R, Suzuki K et al (2013) How occupational health can contribute in a disaster and what we should prepare for the future–lessons learned through support activities of a medical school at the Fukushima Daiichi Nuclear Power Plant in Summer 2011. J Occup Health 55(1):6–10. doi:10.1539/joh.12-0134-CS
Nollet KE (2013) Nollet Q&A with Mayo and ABC. In: Fukushima: lives on the line – a compendium of reports from the 2011 Great East Japan earthquake and tsunami. Minpo, Fukushima, pp 210–213
Ohno K (2010) Risk communication in the medical radiological practice. The 76th seminar of the global strategic centre for radiation health risk control, Nagasaki University, 15 Oct
Royal College of Physicians and Surgeons of Canada (2005) The CanMEDS framework. http://www.royalcollege.ca/portal/page/portal/rc/canmeds/framework. Accessed 5 June 2013
Royal College of Physicians and Surgeons of Canada (2009) Objectives of training in nuclear medicine. Accessed 5 June 2013
Safar P (1974) Critical care medicine – quo vadis? Crit Care Med 2(1):1–5
Starkey J, Maeda S (2011) Earthquake in Japan. Lancet 377(9778):1653. doi:10.1016/S0140-6736(11)60674-0
Staudenherz A, Sinzinger H (2012) "Nuclear" medicine physicians as communicators: their point of view on the aftermath of "nuclear" disaster. Wien Med Wochenschr 162(3–4):60–66
Suzuki Y, Kim Y (2012) The great east Japan earthquake in 2011; toward sustainable mental health care system. Epidemiol Psychiatr Sci 21(1):7–11. doi:10.1017/S2045796011000795
Takeda M (2011) Mental health care and East Japan Great Earthquake. Psychiatry Clin Neurosci 65(3):207–212. doi:10.1111/j.1440-1819.2011.02220.x
Tamura Y, Fukuda K (2011) Earthquake in Japan. Lancet 377(9778):1652. doi:10.1016/S0140-6736(11)60672-7
Tanigawa K, Hosoi Y, Hirohashi N, Iwasaki Y, Kamiya K (2011a) Evacuation from the restricted zone of the damaged Fukushima nuclear power plant: facing with the reality. Resuscitation 82(9):1248. doi:10.1016/j.resuscitation.2011.04.028
Tanigawa K, Hosoi Y, Terasawa S, Kondo H, Asari Y et al (2011b) Lessons learned from the Fukushima Daiichi nuclear power plant accident; the initial 5 days medical activities after the accident. JJAAM 22(9):782–791 (in Japanese)
Tanigawa K, Hosoi Y, Hirohashi N, Iwasaki Y, Kamiya K (2012) Loss of life after evacuation: lessons learned from the Fukushima accident. Lancet 379(9819):889–891. doi:10.1016/S0140-6736(12)60384-5

Tanimoto T, Uchida N, Kodama Y, Teshima T, Taniguchi S (2011) Safety of workers at the Fukushima Daiichi nuclear power plant. Lancet 377(9776):1489–1490. doi:10.1016/S0140-6736(11)60519-9

The Yomiuri Shimbun (2011) Exodus of doctors, nurses adds to Fukushima Prefecture woes. http://www.yomiuri.co.jp/dy/national/T111003004497.htm Accessed 30 May 2012

Wada K, Yoshikawa T, Hayashi T, Aizawa Y (2012) Emergency response technical work at Fukushima Dai-ichi nuclear power plant: occupational health challenges posed by the nuclear disaster. Occup Environ Med 69:599–602. doi:10.1136/oemed-2011-100587

Wolbarst AB, Wiley AL, Nemhauser JB, Christensen DM, Hendee WR (2010) Medical response to a major radiologic emergency: a primer for medical and public health practitioners. Radiology 254(3):660–677

Yasumura S, Goto A, Yamazaki S, Reich MR (2013) Excess mortality among relocated institutionalized elderly after the Fukushima nuclear disaster. Public Health 127(2):186–188. doi:10.1016/j.puhe.2012.10.019

General Considerations in Radiation Disaster Medicine

2

Koichi Tanigawa

Contents

2.1 Introduction 16
2.2 Preparedness and Objectives of Emergency Medicine in Radiation Disaster 16
2.3 Specific Considerations of Radiation Disaster 17
2.4 Basic Knowledge of Radiation 18
2.5 External Exposure and Contamination 20
2.6 Biological Effects of Radiation 21
2.7 Initial Evaluation and Prioritization in Radiation Disaster 23
2.8 Summary 26
References 26

Abstract

Proper understanding on radiation, i.e., types of radiation, effects on humans, and practical measures to protect individuals from radiation, is fundamental in preparation for a radiation disaster. Although a radiation disaster is quite a rare event, medical response shares many aspects in common with other types of disasters. Therefore, effective plans for radiation disaster should be developed within the scope of the general disaster management with specific consideration on radiation in order to develop a sustainable medical response system for this catastrophic event.

K. Tanigawa, M.D., Ph.D.
Department of Emergency and Critical Care Medicine, Hiroshima University, 1-2-3 Kasumi, Minami-ku, Hiroshima 734-8551, Japan
e-mail: tanigawa@hiroshima-u.ac.jp

K. Tanigawa, R.K. Chhem (eds.), *Radiation Disaster Medicine*,
DOI 10.1007/978-3-319-02216-1_2,

© Springer International Publishing Switzerland 2014

2.1 Introduction

Disasters are infrequent, unexpected, and traumatic events that are threatening to social well-being and overwhelming to the coping resources of individuals and communities (Ursano et al. 1994). Disasters interfere with the routines of social life in such a way that extraordinary measures are needed for survival (Porfiriev 1995). Disasters are often classified as natural or man-made; however, the boundaries between the two are blurred when they are defined as the failure of a society to adapt successfully to certain features of its natural and socially constructed environment in a sustainable fashion (Oliver-Smith 1996). A huge earthquake followed by a giant tsunami hit Fukushima prefecture on 11 March 2011. These catastrophic natural events were compounded by a severe accident at the Fukushima Daiichi nuclear power plant creating a tremendous challenge to the Japanese authorities from the disaster management perspectives.

Several radiation accidents of various intensities have occurred in recent history, Chernobyl being the most severe of those events (Linnemann 1987). The most serious events led to overwhelming consequences on individuals and communities because severe radiation accidents generate serious behavioral, physical, and societal impacts with disruption of the preexisting social system. In addition to the fact that radiation carries a negative connotation, any disaster that involves radiation becomes extremely complex to manage especially in terms of public response. Further research by Science and Technology Studies (STS) experts or disaster studies scholars is needed to disentangle the complexity and the implication of accidental radiation effect on society.

A variety of terminology is used to describe accidents that involve radioactive materials and the specific medical response: nuclear accident, radiation emergency, radiation disaster medicine, or nuclear disaster. It is not our purpose to discuss the ontological dimension of the existing terminology. For the purpose of this book, we use "radiation emergency medicine" in the context where the accident can be addressed effectively by a specialized medical team. On the other hand, the term "radiation disaster medicine" is used when the capacity of the medical response team is overwhelmed by the scale of the accident or when its function is disrupted for various reasons.

With this focus in mind, this chapter will present the general purpose of radiation emergency response, radiation protection for the population and workers, and the aim of the various radiation disaster medicine activities in order to effectively integrate efforts in this tragic situation. The involvement of various national and international organizations in medical response and preparedness is covered in Chaps. 5 and 6. The necessity for saving the lives of victims and the protection of the population from ionizing radiation emerges from current knowledge on consequences of disasters, the effects of ionizing radiation on human health, and studies in radiation medicine.

2.2 Preparedness and Objectives of Emergency Medicine in Radiation Disaster

No region in any country in the world is free from the risk of a disaster. Regardless of the magnitude of a disaster such as a major accident (e.g., train crash or terrorist bombing) or a natural disaster (e.g., earthquake and tsunami), medical response in disaster is characterized by the fact that the emergency medical systems are overwhelmed by the expanded medical needs of the sudden number of casualties. Therefore, infrastructure and functional requirements for disaster have been developed at national as well as local levels in most countries.

Contrary to the public conception, most of the medical needs required in a radiation disaster are quite similar to other types of disaster (Protasova et al. 1997; Tanigawa et al. 2012; Wada et al. 2012). In addition, the rarity of the event makes it difficult to develop a sustainable emergency medical response system solely applicable to radiation disaster. We therefore emphasize that medical management for radiation disaster should be integrated into the scope of general disaster management. The system should not be developed separately from general disaster planning, with an emphasis on the optimal utilization of medical resources. In addition, the specific considerations of radiation disaster must be applied.

2.3 Specific Considerations of Radiation Disaster

Major radiological events in radiation disasters include severe nuclear reactor accidents or nuclear explosions. When a radiation disaster occurs, information is usually scarce and/or becomes intricate and may not be provided in a timely fashion. Sophisticated radiological survey systems may not give accurate data due to power failure and/or structural damages to the system or monitoring posts. Due to the impacts of radiation, local emergency medical systems may not be able to cope with mass casualty events (MCE) such as results from an explosion. During evacuation, residents may not observe proper protection from radiation in their rush to leave. Some of the hospitals and nursing care facilities in the evacuation zone may become isolated and hence become unable to provide appropriate care for patients because of shortage of food, medical supplies, and medical personnel. Unplanned evacuation of these patients may pose a significant health risk to them, such as was the case in Fukushima (Tanigawa et al. 2012; The National Diet of Japan 2012).

Levels of care provided in radiation disasters rely on the functional local and national emergency medical system. The impact of radiation can jeopardize the local medical response systems when medical needs increase. In situations where evacuation is mandated, additional medical needs arise for evacuation of patients in hospitals and the elderly in care facilities. With these considerations, the disaster plan should dictate the utilization of all available resources to prevent further casualties in each phase of the radiation disaster.

The objectives of radiation disaster medicine are to maximize the chance of survival of the most persons who are faced with life-threatening conditions, to prevent or reduce deterministic health effects, to reasonably reduce risk of stochastic effects, and to mitigate psychological impact.

Personnel involved in such activities should acquire basic understanding of radiation with regard to human health. Proper understanding will help to organize the activities of the emergency medical response in the most efficient way while minimizing radiation risk to all individuals involved.

2.4 Basic Knowledge of Radiation

Radiation exists in all places that we live. Humans and animals are exposed to natural radiation from cosmic waves, which are radioactive materials in nature. We eat food containing natural radioactive potassium and carbon, which stay in our body. In modern societies, radiation is widely used for energy production, industry, medicine, and the military. As medical professionals, we utilize radiation in diagnosis and treatment for various types of injury and disease such as cancer, cardiovascular diseases, and trauma. However, we usually do not recognize how close we are to radiation in our daily life.

Radiation is a flow of energy that travels through the air and collides with substances resulting in changes to these substances by transferring some energy to them, by removing tightly bound electrons from atoms, thus creating ions. This phenomenon is called ionization; therefore, this type of radiation is precisely called ionizing radiation. On the other hand, light, ultraviolet light, and waves of mobile phones do not have enough energy to ionize atoms or molecules; therefore, they are not ionizing radiation. Alpha particles consist of two protons and two neutrons bound together into a particle identical to a helium nucleus. Beta particles are high-energy, high-speed electrons. Beta particles emitted are as a form of ionizing radiation also known as beta rays.

Radioactive materials are physically unstable and decay into more stable materials when they emit radiation. Although there are a number of radioactive materials, only several types of radiation exist (Fig. 2.1). Radiation includes a particle or an electromagnetic wave: alpha particles, beta particles, gamma ray, X-ray, and neutrons. Radioactive materials such as uranium and plutonium give off alpha particles when they decay. Radioactive iodine-131 (^{131}I) and radioactive cesium-137 (^{137}Cs), which are the major radioactive materials released in a nuclear reactor accident, emit beta particles as well as gamma rays. Radioactive strontium-90 (^{90}Sr), which was found in the soil and water near Fukushima Daiichi nuclear power plant (NPP), emits beta particles. Radioactive cobalt-60 (^{60}Co) is also found in a NPP accident.

Radiation has unique characteristics in terms of travel and penetrating through other substances. The ability to penetrate varies between radiation types (Fig. 2.1). Alpha and beta particles only travel for a very limited distance. Alpha particles do not penetrate much (travel only a few centimeters in the air) and can be blocked with a single sheet of paper. Beta particles are more penetrating than alpha particles; however, they can be blocked with a few millimeters thick of aluminum sheet. Although they have relatively weak penetrating features, alpha and beta radiations give high amounts of energy to tissues resulting in serious damage if incorporated into the body.

On the other hand, gamma rays are very penetrative and easily travel through thin lead aprons commonly used for protection from X-ray energies used in medical imaging. In Fukushima (especially at the damaged nuclear power plant), there are places with extremely high gamma radiation levels which gamma rays accounted for. A thick concrete block or lead wall is required to block gamma rays. Neutrons are extremely penetrating; they can only be stopped by thick masses of concrete,

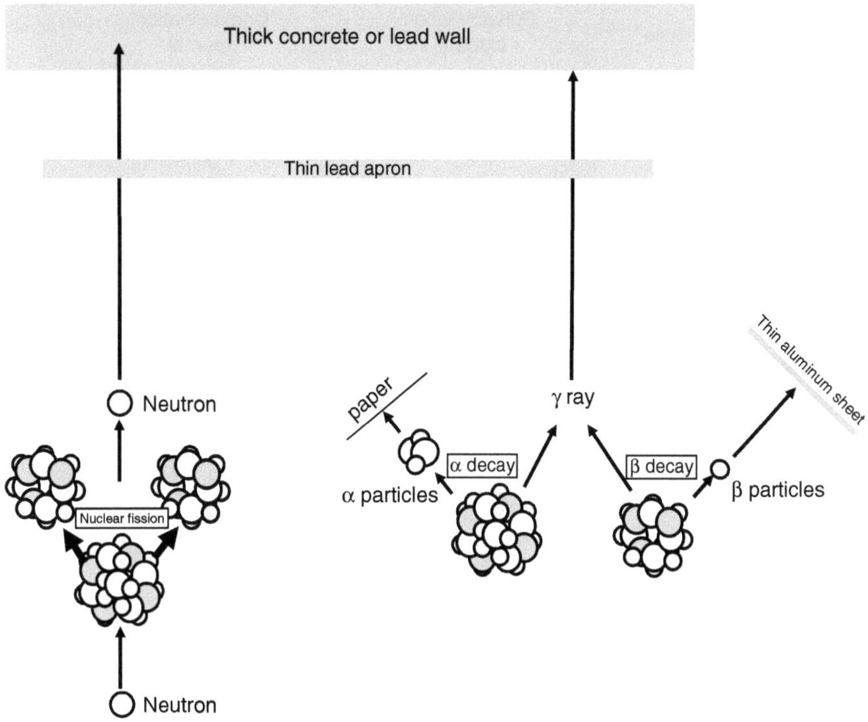

Fig. 2.1 Radionuclides and radiations

water, or paraffin. In addition, neutrons have a unique feature of inducing radioactivity when absorbed by stable materials. Neutrons are produced mostly in a specific condition called nuclear fission which takes place inside nuclear reactors in operation or in a nuclear detonation. In the JCO Co. Ltd. Tokai Plant accident, three workers were exposed to very high levels of neutrons which were produced in a nuclear fission induced while they were dissolving U_3O_8 (18.8 % enriched) and pouring nitrate solution into a precipitation vessel using a funnel. External exposure was the major health problem (IAEA 2000).

The toxicity of a radioactive material depends on the type of radiation emitted, physical and biological half-life, target organs, and toxic natures of the substance itself. Toxicity of radiation is modified by linear energy transfer (LET), which is a measure of how much energy is transferred from ionizing radiation to tissue. Alpha particles and neutrons have high LET, whereas gamma rays and X-rays have low LET. For example, ^{131}I has a short half-life of 8 days. However, ^{131}I has a strong affinity to the thyroid gland, staying in the tissue while emitting beta particles which may result in later development of cancer. Another example is ^{137}Cs that has a relatively long half-life of 30 years; however, the biological half-life is 9 days in small children and approximately 109 days for adults. Cesium acts like potassium, spreading throughout the body after incorporation and is excreted into urine. Plutonium-239 (^{239}Pu) inhaled

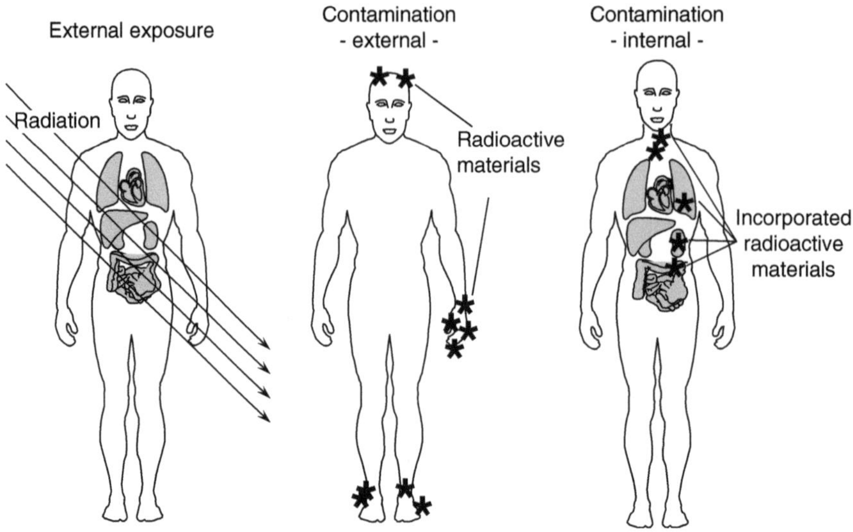

Fig. 2.2 External exposure and contamination

into the lung moves to the bone and liver, resulting in damage to these organs through the effects of alpha particles over many years. The effects of radiation are broadly divided into two types: external exposure and contamination (Fig. 2.2).

2.5 External Exposure and Contamination

External exposure means being exposed to radiation from the outside of the body. Individuals who are externally exposed to radiation have not absorbed any radioactive substances and are therefore not "radioactive." In the Fukushima accident, gamma rays emitted from ^{131}I in the early phase and ^{137}Cs in the late phase after the accident were major sources of external exposure.

Contamination takes place internally and/or externally. Internal contamination refers to a status where radioactive materials are incorporated into the body. With internal contamination, the substance may stay in the body for a certain period of time depending on the physical and biological half-life of the substance, and during this time they exert an effect on tissues and organs because of the deposited radiation sources.

The mode of internal contamination is through inhalation, digestion, and absorption from open wounds of the skin. In the Fukushima accident, the highest level of radiation exposure for workers was 678 mSv (Sv: Sievert, unit of irradiation which the body is exposed) of which internal contamination accounted for 590 mSv (The National Diet of Japan 2012). The entry of radioactive materials into the body was mostly through inhalation because it was found later that this worker did not wear effective face masks. The legal radiation exposure for a rescue worker was raised from 100 to 250 mSv on 15 March 2011 (The National Diet of Japan 2012). In the Chernobyl accident, on the other hand, local residents including small children were

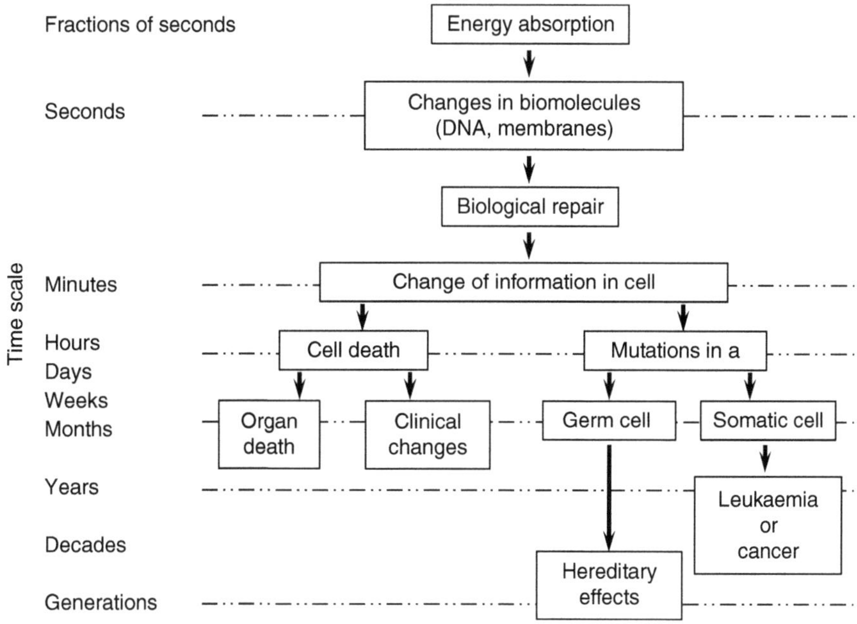

Fig. 2.3 Effects of radiation

exposed internally by taking dairy products contaminated with radioactive iodine-131 (^{131}I), resulting in a high incidence of thyroid cancer (The Chernobyl Forum 2006).

External contamination refers to a status where radioactive materials such as radioactive dusts or particulates get attached to the skin or clothes. In this case, the body is exposed to radiation from outside the body, and it carries a high risk of internal contamination by accidental inhalation, ingestion, or absorption of deposited radioactive materials. In the Fukushima accident, most of the severe contamination observed among workers was through exposure to contaminated water. Two workers became contaminated on their feet by immersion in heavily contaminated water in the No. 3 reactor building. Also, radioactive dust or plume released after Fukushima accident contaminated thousands of residents (The National Diet of Japan 2012).

2.6 Biological Effects of Radiation

Living cells undergo divisions vigorously to create new cells. The DNA of the cell has genetic information and is essential for cell division. Beyond a certain level of radiation exposure, the cell membrane and cyto-cellular DNA are damaged. Because genetic material is particularly sensitive to radiation, tissues that divide rapidly (such as bone marrow and intestinal cells) are more sensitive to damage than those with slower cell divisions (such as muscle and neuron) (Fig. 2.3) (IAEA 2002). Natural radiation does exist, to which we are constantly exposed in our daily life. Our body has protective mechanisms to reduce the effects of radiation. However, if

Table 2.1 The effects of radiation on humans (Saito 2012)

Dose exposed	Effects on individuals	Consequences of a group exposed
Less than 10 mSv	No acute effects Minimum increased risk for cancer	No increase in incidence of cancer
10–100 mSv	No acute effects Less than 1 % increased risk for cancer	Possible increase in incidence of cancer in a group greater than 100,000 population
100–1,000 mSv	Acute effects 10 % increased risk for cancer	Probable increase in incidence of cancer in a group of a few millions population
Greater than 1,000 mSv	Acute effects, death Substantial increased risk for cancer	Increase in incidence of cancer

the exposure dose of radiation exceeds the levels such that the protective mechanisms do not work anymore, acute radiation effects take place, which is called the deterministic effects (Fig. 2.3).

Acute effects consist of whole body and local injuries. Acute radiation exposure of the whole body greater than 1 Sv leads to loss of appetite, nausea, vomiting, and diarrhea (these syndromes are called prodromal signs). Radiation injuries to the bone marrow result in pancytopenia and predisposition to bleeding diathesis and infection within 1 or 2 weeks. Gastrointestinal symptoms also ensue following exposure. These symptoms are called acute radiation syndrome (see Chap. 3). Regarding local effects, most of them are dermatological injuries. Although radiation dermatitis is often called radiation burn, the mechanisms involved are quite different from thermal burn. Depending on the different sensitivities of the cells of the dermis to radiation, various pathological changes such as redness (initial erythema), edema, bulla formation, erosion, and ulceration ensue. It takes weeks to develop radiation dermal injuries.

As for long-term effects of radiation, when the DNA of certain tissues is exposed to radiation, cancer can develop as a late effect (Fig. 2.3). In this instance, the DNA injured by radiation is incorporated into the genes as a mutation, resulting in the tissues becoming malignant in the future. This is called the stochastic effect.

The effects of radiation on human are summarized in Table 2.1 (Saito 2012). The International Commission on Radiological Protection (ICRP) has advised the safety levels of radiation exposure for occupational limits be less than 100 mSv over 5 years (average permitted exposure less than 20 mSv per year), not exceeding 50 mSv per year (Fig. 2.4) (ICRP 1991). In the Fukushima accident, the upper limit of alarm was set at 30 mSv for rescue and fire department personnel (The local nuclear emergency response headquarters of Fukushima Daiichi Nuclear Power Plant Accident 2011). However, the ICRP recommends reference levels of 500–1,000 mSv to avoid the occurrence of severe deterministic injuries for rescue workers involved in an emergency exposure situation. This means that it will be justified to expend significant resources, both at the planning stage and during the response,

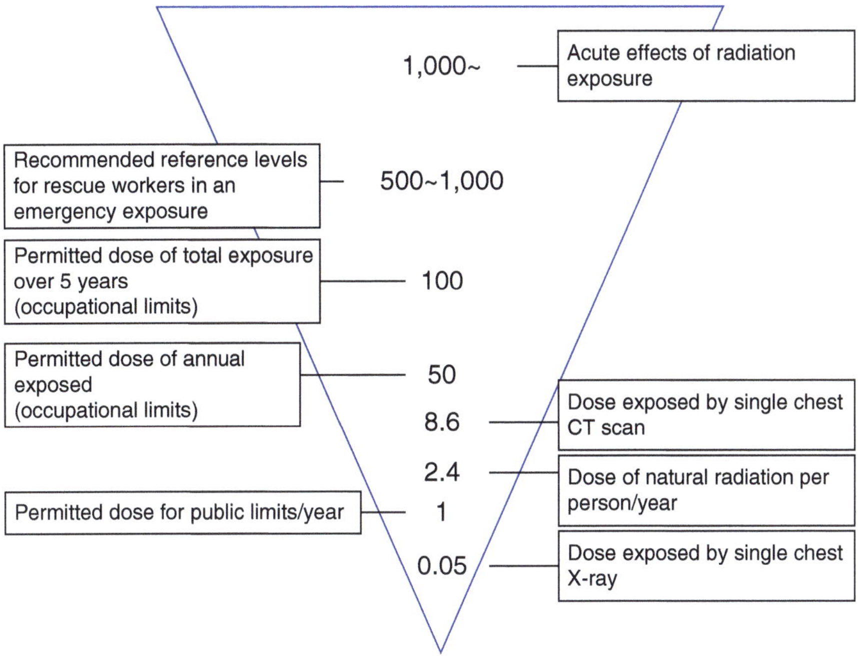

Fig. 2.4 Permitted dose exposure and reference levels (unit: mSv)

if required, in order to reduce expected exposures to below these levels. Furthermore, the ICRP recommends no dose restrictions for lifesaving efforts by informed volunteers if the benefit to others outweighs the rescuer's risk (ICRP 2007, 2009).

2.7 Initial Evaluation and Prioritization in Radiation Disaster

Major radiation hazards in radiation disaster are radioactive dusts and plume. Radioactive plume does not spread in a concentric fashion. It spreads while quickly changing its direction due to the wind direction, geographic features, and weather conditions. Frequent monitoring of ambient dose rate is required by, for example, considering the effect of the wind direction and planning an approach from a windward side.

In disasters, marked difficulties arise in coping with expanded medical needs, while available resources are limited. Under these circumstances, the priority has to be put on victims with higher chances of survival with any types of life-threatening conditions. Trauma is the major cause of death in disaster, therefore, criteria for triage has been developed by focusing on preventable death from trauma. On the other hand, radiation is not a cause of immediate life-threatening conditions and death. In addition, emergency medical needs such as trauma and acute illnesses have been the

Table 2.2 Major points in the initial evaluation of the victim

Four major points in initial evaluation	Examples
1. Look for causes other than radiation if victims are unconscious, disoriented, burned, or otherwise in distress, such as trauma, chemical injuries, or illnesses	At the time of the JCO accident in Japan, three workers were exposed to a high dose, and regrettably two of them died. But even though it was a considerable exposure dose, they did not die soon after it In the Fukushima Daiichi nuclear power plant accident, four workers died during restoration activities, but that was due to acute myocardial infarction or sepsis During emergency evacuation, hospital patients and the elderly died because of deterioration of underlying medical problems, hypothermia, or dehydration
2. No risk for the medical personnel providing aid to a person exposed to radiation from external sources	Patient who received chest X-ray or CT is never radioactive
3. Very limited health risk to medical personnel in treating a person externally contaminated with radioactive materials if the victim's contaminated clothes are removed and replaced with non-contaminated clothes or sheets	No radiation accident victims – including all those at Goiania, Brazil, in 1987 – have ever presented a threat to responders and medical personnel The only exception was a case of a few Chernobyl victims who were extremely severely contaminated with radioactive aerosols and thus exposed the medical personnel to some radiation
4. No harm or direct hazard to any other person from an internally contaminated individual	The doses of radioactive iodine incorporated into the body in the Chernobyl or Fukushima accident were far less than the radiation levels at which the patient is allowed to be discharged after receiving a massive dose of radioactive iodine for thyroid cancer

major health hazards in the reported radiation disasters. Therefore, the same approaches as other type of disasters can be applied in a radiation disaster with the addition of specific management for radiation exposure.

In the initial evaluation of the patient, several points need to be addressed (Table 2.2) (IAEA 2005). Firstly, exposure to radiation does not immediately cause life-threatening conditions immediately postexposure. If victims are unconscious, disoriented, burned, or otherwise in distress, look for causes other than radiation. Secondly, medical responders must be aware that a person who was exposed externally has no radiation threat whatsoever to them. Thirdly, there is very limited health risk to medical personnel in treating a person with external contamination if the victim's contaminated clothes are removed. Fourthly, an individual contaminated internally does not present any harm or direct hazard to any other person.

Radiation cannot be seen nor felt. However, radiation can be measured or monitored easily with devices such as Geiger-Mueller (GM) survey meters, NaI scintillation survey meters, or ionizing chamber survey meters (Table 2.3). By using these

Table 2.3 Survey meters used for measurement of radiation

Survey meters	Radiation detected
GM survey meter The most common device used for the detection of surface contamination	Beta particles and gamma rays
NaI scintillation survey meter Used for dose rate measurement with unit of microSv/h, sensitive at lower dose rate	Gamma rays
Ionizing chamber survey meter Used to measure at higher dose rate (up to 1 Sv/hr)	Gamma rays

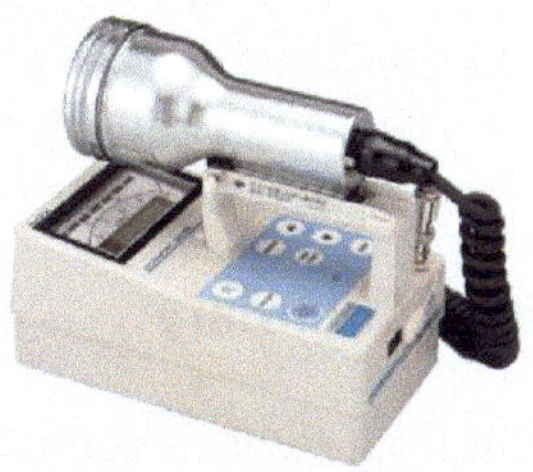

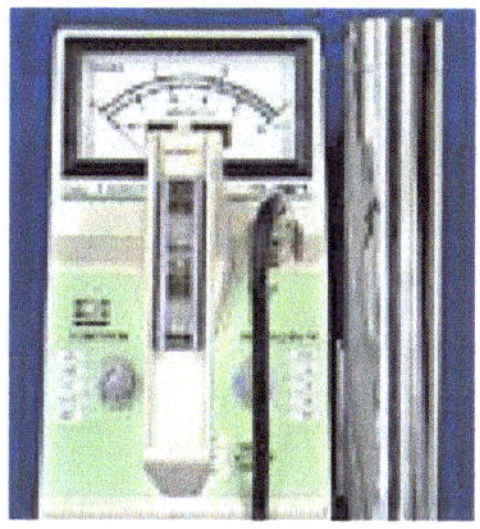

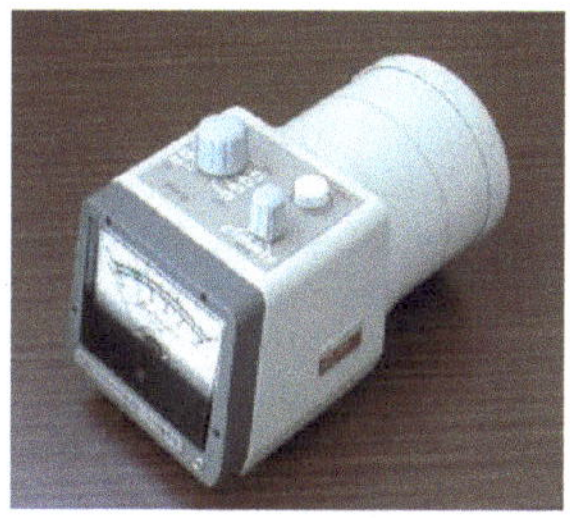

devices properly, one can identify the area contaminated and conduct real-time measurement of the levels of radiation.

ALARA stands for "As Low As Reasonably Achievable," meaning making every reasonable effort to maintain exposures to radiation as far below as the regulatory dose limits as practical, taking into account economic, societal, and other relevant considerations (Lochard 2009). Although the ALARA principle cannot be applied appropriately in such a harsh condition as radiation disaster, one should make efforts to minimize effects of radiation by minimizing the time spent near the radiation source, maximizing the distance away from the radiation source, making use of shielding for reduction of external radiation, and minimizing and controlling contamination with properly use of protective clothing and equipment.

The principle of the emergency medical approaches to the patient in radiation disaster is, therefore, the same as that applied for other types of disasters or regular emergency cases; treat the life-threatening injuries first. Triage criteria such as START (Simple Triage and Rapid Treatment) (Benson et al. 1996) should come first as advanced trauma life support for trauma victims and advanced cardiovascular life support for patients with acute cardiovascular diseases being prioritized over the examination and treatment of radiation injury/effects.

2.8 Summary

Medical approaches required in a radiation disaster have many aspects in common with other types of disasters. With proper understanding of radiation, one will be able to establish effective plans within the scope of the general disaster management, to better prepare for effective use of preexisting resources, and to provide appropriate medical care for victims in a very difficult situation such as in a radiation disaster.

Acknowledgments The author would like to thank Dr. Kazuhiko Maekawa and Dr. Penelope Engel-Hills for their editorial assistance and valuable input.

References

Benson M, Koenig KL, Schultz CH (1996) Disaster triage: START, then SAVE – a new method of dynamic triage for victims of a catastrophic earthquake. Prehospital Disaster Med 11: 117–124

International Atomic Energy Agency (2000) IAEA reports on Tokaimura accident. International Atomic Energy Agency. Health Phys 78(2):231

International Atomic Energy Agency (2002) Dose-effect curves; deterministic and stochastic effects of radiation, module IX. In: Emergency preparedness and response: medical preparedness and response, EPR-MEDICAL-T. IAEA, Vienna

International Atomic Energy Agency (2005) Generic procedures for medical response during a nuclear or radiological emergency. EPR-MEDICAL. IAEA, Vienna

International Commission on Radiological Protection (1991) 1990 recommendation of the international commission on radiological protection. Ann ICRP 21(1–3):52–66

International Commission on Radiological Protection (2007) The 2007 recommendations of the international commission on radiological protection. ICRP publication 103. Ann ICRP 37(2–4):103–122

International Commission on Radiological Protection (2009) Application of the Commission's recommendations for the protection of people in emergency exposure situations. ICRP publication 109. Ann ICRP 39(1):1–110

Linnemann RE (1987) Soviet medical response to the Chernobyl nuclear accident. JAMA 257(5):637–643

Lochard J (2009) ALARA in safety and security of radiation sources: an ICRP perspective. Paper presented at the 12th European ALARA network workshop, Vienna, 21–23 Oct 2009

Oliver-Smith A (1996) Anthropological research on hazards and disasters. Ann Rev Anthropol 25:303–328

Porfiriev BN (1995) Disaster and disaster areas: methodological issues of definition and delineation. Int J Mass Emerg Disaster 13(3):285–304

Protasova TG, Leliuk VG, Gus'kova AK (1997) Causes of death of persons exposed to health hazards in the area of the Chernobyl accident. Klin Med (Mosk) 75(11):41–47 (in Russian)
Saito T (2012) How to explain the effects of radiation exactly to your patients? Nippon Rinsho 70(3):362–365 (in Japanese)
Tanigawa K, Hosoi Y, Hirohashi N, Iwasaki Y, Kamiya K (2012) Loss of life after evacuation: lessons learned from the Fukushima accident. Lancet 379(10):889–891
The Chernobyl Forum (2006) Chernobyl's legacy: health, environmental and socio-economic impacts and recommendations to the governments of Belarus, the Russian Federation and Ukraine. 2003–2005 IAEA, Vienna. http://www.iaea.org/Publications/Booklets/Chernobyl/chernobyl.pdf. Accessed 2 Apr 2013
The local nuclear emergency response headquarters of Fukushima Daiichi Nuclear Power Plant Accident (2011) Management plan for injured individuals in accidents. Notification as of April 2nd (in Japanese)
The National Diet of Japan (2012) The official report of. The Fukushima Nuclear Accident Independent Investigation Commission: executive summary, The National Diet of Japan, Japan
Ursano RJ, McCaughey BG, Fullerton C (1994) Individual and community responses to disaster: the structure of human chaos. Cambridge University Press, Cambridge, UK
Wada K, Yoshikawa T, Hayashi T, Aizawa Y (2012) Emergency response technical work at Fukushima Daichi nuclear power plant: occupational health challenges posed by the nuclear disaster. Occup Environ Med 69(8):599–602. doi:10.1136/oemed-2011-100587

Medical Perspective

3

Koichi Tanigawa and Arifumi Hasegawa

Contents

3.1 Prehospital Emergency Medical Response 30
3.1.1 Introduction 30
3.1.2 Reestablishment of a Medical Response System in the Region 30
3.1.3 Establishment of a Command Center 40
3.1.4 Information on Radiation 41
3.1.5 Development of a Sustainable Local Emergency Medical System 42
3.1.6 Major Public Health Consequences Following Evacuation 44
3.1.7 Summary 46
3.1.8 Experiences from the Initial Medical Response in Fukushima Accident 46
3.2 Hospital Emergency Medical Response 58
3.2.1 Introduction 58
3.2.2 Planning 58
3.2.3 General Considerations of Hospital Response 60
3.2.4 Hospital Emergency Response 60
3.2.5 Dose Assessment 68
3.2.6 Local Radiation Injury (LRI) 68
3.2.7 Acute Radiation Syndrome (ARS) 68
3.2.8 Summary 72
3.2.9 Experiences from Fukushima Accident 72
References 76

K. Tanigawa, M.D., Ph.D. (✉)
Department of Emergency and Critical Care Medicine, Hiroshima University,
1-2-3 Kasumi, Minami-ku, Hiroshima 734-8551, Japan
e-mail: tanigawa@hiroshima-u.ac.jp

A. Hasegawa, M.D., Ph.D.
Department of Emergency and Critical Care Medicine,
Radiation Disaster Medical Center, Fukushima Medical University, 1 Hikarigaoka,
Fukushima 960-1295, Japan
e-mail: hase@fmu.ac.jp

K. Tanigawa, R.K. Chhem (eds.), *Radiation Disaster Medicine*,
DOI 10.1007/978-3-319-02216-1_3, © Springer International Publishing Switzerland 2014

3.1 Prehospital Emergency Medical Response

Koichi Tanigawa

Abstract

The impacts of radiation disaster on society are so deep that important elements of the medical response system including prehospital emergency care may be lost. Expanded medical needs for evacuation of inpatients or mass casualty events may occur simultaneously. In addition, displacement of hundreds of thousands of citizens may pose serious public healthcare issues. Not only medical resources for general disasters should be maximally utilized, but also all available resources from other regions across the nation should be mobilized to strengthen the medical response system in the affected regions. A sustainable emergency medical and public healthcare system should be established to counteract the long lasting impacts of radiation disaster.

3.1.1 Introduction

The biggest challenge in a radiation disaster is the loss of important elements of the medical response system due to the impacts of radiation. Thousands of workers, fire fighters, and military personnel are mobilized to engage in the restoration activities, and evacuation of residents is urgently performed, while the local emergency medical response system may lose its ability to function effectively. The specific features of a radiation disaster are characterized as follows:

1. The local emergency medical system is partially or completely lost because of the impact of radiation.
2. Release of massive doses of radioactive materials makes it difficult to set up any safety zone for the command center near the disaster site.
3. Radiation dose monitoring systems may not work, and information on radiation may not be available in a timely fashion.
4. It usually takes an extended time period to ensure that the damaged facility is under control. In the early phase, severe acute radiation syndrome may be encountered, and isolated trauma cases or severe acute radiation illnesses, with or without contamination, are frequently observed during this period.
5. Displaced people may have to stay in shelters or other places for months or even years. This can lead to severe public healthcare issues.

3.1.2 Reestablishment of a Medical Response System in the Region

Soon after the accident, the local medical system, including the emergency medical services system, may not function properly due to the risks of radiation and the designation of an evacuation zone. At this stage, a mass casualty event (MCE) in the accident site may occur, and hospital patients and/or elderly persons in care facilities may commence with evacuation. In Fukushima, not only all hospitals and care facilities in the region but also the primary radiation emergency medical hospitals were forced to close because of the evacuation order (see Sect. 3.1.8). Hundreds of hospital patients and elderly persons at care facilities were hurriedly transported out from the evacuation zone. Exactly at the same time, an explosion occurred at the nuclear power plant. This was the moment when the medical needs suddenly expanded. In that sense, an emergency medical response in a radiation disaster is quite similar to that in other types of major disasters such as a huge earthquake.

3.1.2.1 Planning for Medical Responses in an MCE and Evacuation of Inpatients

The role of each component of the emergency response system, i.e., the nuclear facility, fire departments, police, hospitals, military, and the local and national government must be determined during advance planning. The focus should be on field care and patient triage; decontamination, transportation, and distribution; and hospital-based acute care and treatment for radiation injuries. Also, protocols for secondary transfer to other facilities out of the disaster region and methods of transportation should be drawn up. Ideally, medical advisers who are familiar with the local emergency medical system, and specialize not only in radiation emergency medicine but also disaster medicine, should be designated in planning. In the event of a radiation disaster, these medical advisers will join the command center to coordinate the activities (Morimura et al. 2012).

In evacuation planning, essentials that need consideration include distribution of hospitals and care facilities, number of patients in the area, available vehicles, evacuation routes, estimated time for evacuation, and available hospitals and facilities for evacuees (Yamamoto 1993). Medical teams should be mobilized to attend to the patients for evacuation. The role of the medical team will start before evacuation, as proper care may not have been provided for patients, due to the establishment of the restricted zone. Therefore, the medical team should triage patients, provide medical care as needed before evacuation, and arrange appropriate methods of transportation (Fig. 3.1). If possible, medical care should be continued during and after evacuation. The medical team, consisting of doctors, nurses, technologists for radiological examinations, and logistics personnel, should be trained for a radiation emergency and be appropriately equipped with necessary items such as personal protective equipment (PPE) and radiation meters.

Reestablishment of a medical response system in a radiation disaster should be planned in advance. Based on the simulated spread patterns of contaminated areas and available medical resources, i.e., hospitals, fire departments, and access, several alternative plans should be determined.

In the event of a disaster, establish a medical response system as soon as possible to prepare for MCE and evacuation. In accord with the plan, mobilize all available regional and national resources to the area to strengthen the local medical response system. In order to achieve these goals, local authorities as well as the national government must understand the consequences of a radiation disaster and make plans

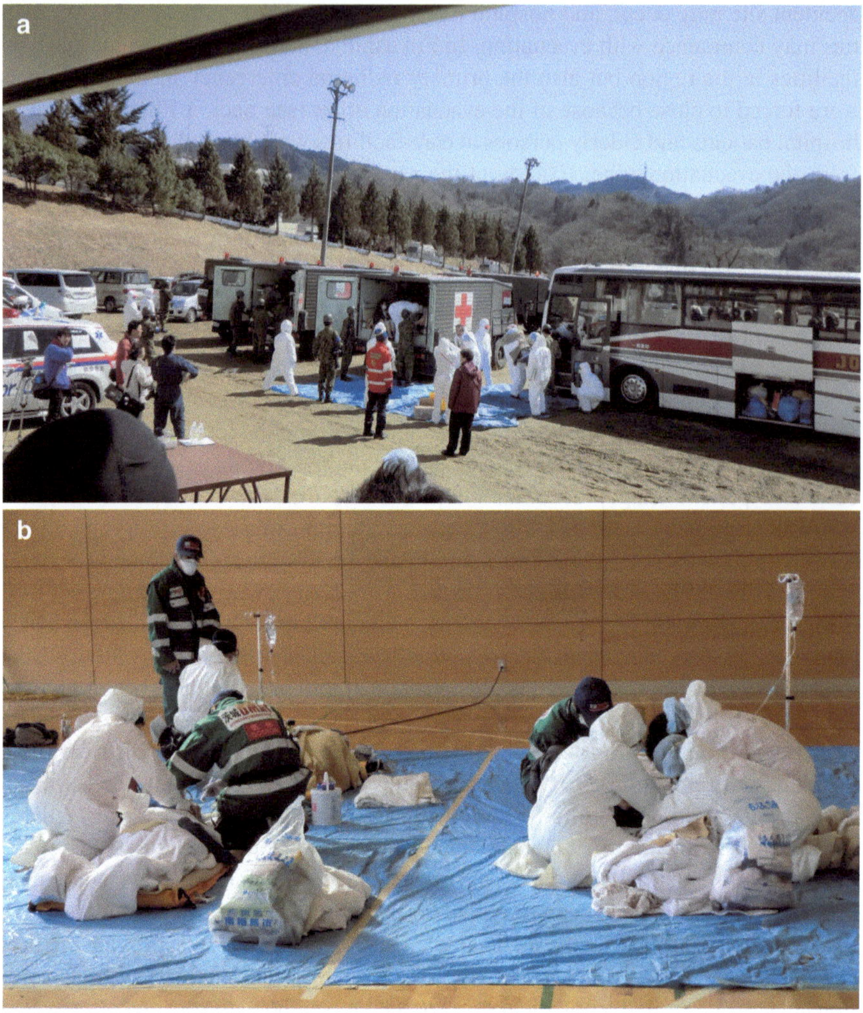

Fig. 3.1 Evacuation of inpatients supported by Disaster Medical Assistance Teams (DMATs). Ambulances and Japan Self-Defense Force (JSDF) vehicles were mobilized to the collection area (*upper photo*). Patients were triaged and provided care before transportation (*lower photo*)

to reestablish an emergency medical response system suited for the specific medical needs in the region.

3.1.2.2 General Concepts in Prehospital Emergency Response

Although a radiation disaster is quite rare, its effects will be devastating not only for the individuals but also for the whole society and the nation. However, most of the medical resources required in a radiation disaster can be provided with structural and functional resources for disaster medicine with specific requirements for protection from radiation. Proper understanding of radiation is fundamental to

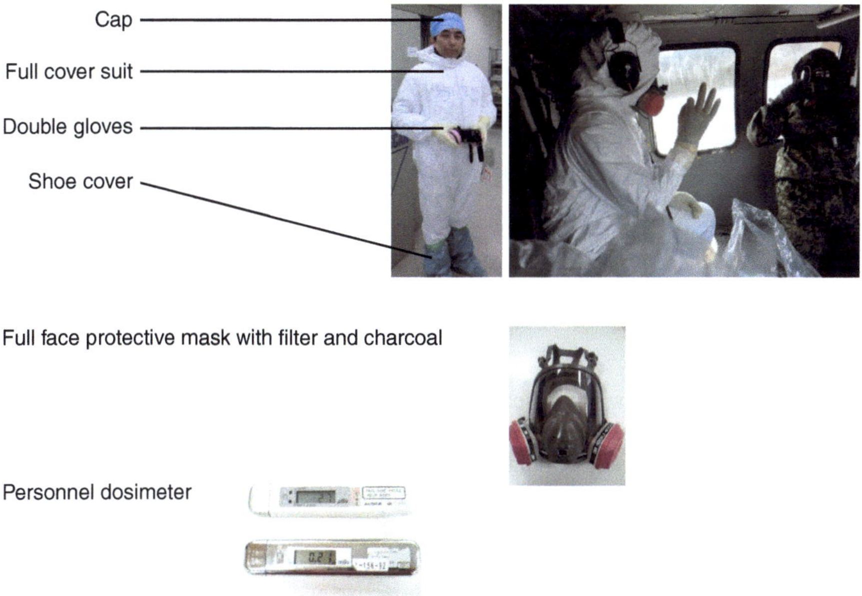

Fig. 3.2 Personal protective equipment (PPE) required for field missions

saving the lives of victims as well as minimizing the effects of radiation on the rescuers and victims.

3.1.2.2.1 Basic Understanding Required for Medical Response

Radiation effects on individuals can be from external and/or internal dose. Emergency personnel should always keep in mind the basic principle of protection from external radiation: distance, time, and shield. Also, they should avoid internal contamination (refer to Chap. 2). By observing the basic principle of protection, one can control the effects of radiation.

Initial information is usually very scarce in radiation disasters as with other types of disasters. In any situation where involvement of radioactive materials is suspected, absorption of radioactive materials should be minimized as much as possible by wearing personal protective equipment (PPE) with an effective mask for radioactive materials (Fig. 3.2). The full face mask should be checked for appropriate filters and/or charcoal before use and no leak must be observed when the mask is put on the face. By using radiation survey meters and a personal dosimeter, one can determine radiation doses and estimate how much individuals are exposed to externally.

Until involved radioactive materials are determined, one can anticipate the most likely sources of radiation based on information of the site, types of operation, and nature of the accident (Table 3.1) (International Atomic Energy Agency [IAEA] 2002a). For example, in a nuclear accident, radioactive iodine (^{131}I, ^{133}I) and cesium (^{137}Cs, ^{134}Cs), besides radioactive gases, i.e., ^{85}Kr and ^{133}Xe, are likely to be released

Table 3.1 Types of radiation accidents, effects, and major source of dose

Accident	Critical organ	Major source of dose
Reactors (power, research, ship)	Whole body (bone marrow)	Gamma
	Skin	Beta
	Thyroid	Radioiodine
Spent reactor fuel storage or reprocessing	Whole body (bone marrow)	Gamma
Industrial and medical gamma sources (sealed)	Whole body (bone marrow)	Gamma
	Skin	Gamma
Industrial and medical gamma sources (damaged, unsealed)	Whole body (bone marrow)	Gamma
	Skin	Beta
Pu – weapons damage or manufacture	Lung	Alpha

into the atmosphere when a nuclear fuel container is breached during the operation of a nuclear reactor. In addition, heavy metals such as ^{90}Sr and ^{239}Pu might contaminate soil or water adjacent to a damaged reactor.

The effects of radiation after a nuclear reactor accident are mainly due to released radioactive vapors, dust, and nuclear fallout (the radioactive particles that fall to the ground, trees, grass, or buildings). High levels of ambient radiation are mainly due to gamma rays emitted from released radioactive materials. In emergency situations, the International Commission on Radiological Protection (ICRP) (2007) sets no dose restrictions for saving lives if and only if the benefit to others clearly outweighs the rescuer's own risk. To prevent the development of catastrophic situations, radiation exposure for emergency personnel must not exceed the range from 500 mSv up to 1,000 mSv in order to avoid acute radiation injuries.

Among radioactive materials released in a nuclear reactor accident, ^{131}I and ^{137}Cs are the major health hazards. In addition to wearing PPE, those who are younger than 40 years old will be advised to take potassium iodide (KI) to prevent deposition of radioactive iodine in the thyroid gland. When the use of KI is indicated, it should be prepared prior to the field mission. The indicated level of weighted, committed dose equivalent to the thyroid is 50–100 mSv (IAEA 2011). However, in a field mission, estimation of thyroid doses is quite difficult and impracticable. Therefore, prophylactic administration of KI is recommended for those who are about to engage in activities in an environment where large doses of radioactive iodine is likely to be released.

Persian blue (PB) is indicated in case of radioactive cesium absorption. PB is an inert medication and expected to block the reabsorption process in the small intestine.

Experiences from Fukushima Accident: At 6 am on 15 March 2011, the No. 4 reactor building exploded and the No. 2 reactor building was severely damaged. Following these events, the radiation level reached its peak at 9 am on the same day, which was 11,930 μSv/h at the main gate, 900 m west from the damaged reactor building in Fukushima Daiichi nuclear power plant (NPP) (The National Diet of Japan 2012). On 16 March, we flew from Fukushima Medical University to pick up a worker who sustained chest injury and contamination at Fukushima Daini NPP. To reduce the effects of radiation, we wore PPE, monitored dose rate, and minimized the time of stay on the site. Figure 3.3 shows the time we left Fukushima Medical University at

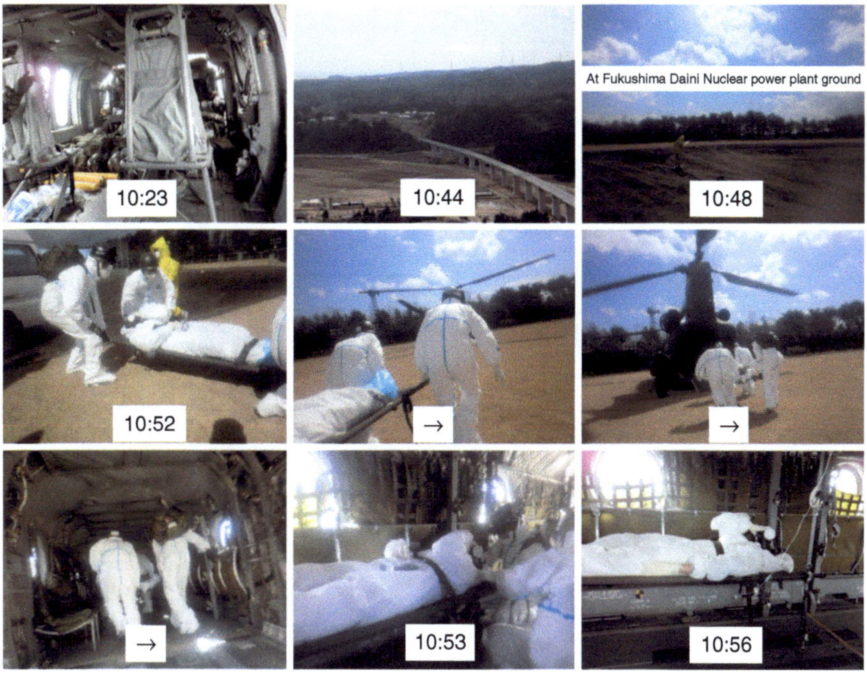

Fig. 3.3 Reducing time in the field to minimize radiation exposure

10:23 (upper left), arrived at the site (10:48), picked up the worker (10:52), moved into the helicopter (10:53), and left the site. By limiting the time, the total exposure dose was controlled to 12 μSv, one quarter of the dose of a single chest X-ray.

3.1.2.2.2 Goals of Prehospital Emergency Medical Response

In a radiation disaster, the main goals of prehospital emergency medical response are:

1. To manage the on-site response taking specific features in a radiation disaster into consideration
2. To triage victims in order to maximize the survival of the most who are facing with life-threatening conditions
3. To treat injuries resulting from an emergency situation and radiation exposure

Management of On-Site Response in Radiation Disaster

When a radiation disaster occurs, the restricted area is established soon and only authorized personnel are allowed to enter. Therefore, the facility personnel who have been adequately trained in techniques of radiological survey, rescue, and basic life support are to provide emergency first aid for injured persons until emergency responders from the fire department arrive.

Due to the effects of radiation, the safety zone where victims are collected, triaged, and treated in case of MCE may not be available nearby (National Center for Injury Prevention and Control 2010). In addition, wearing PPE makes it quite difficult for rescue personnel to communicate, perform triage, and provide first aid in

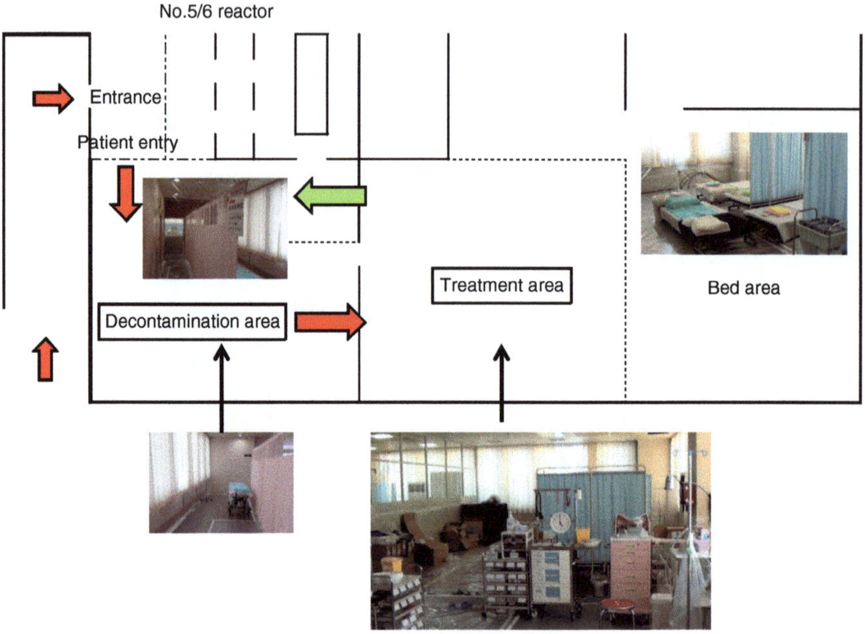

Fig. 3.4 Example of an in-house decontamination and treatment area (the emergency room of Fukushima Daiichi NPP)

the field. In the first explosion that took place on 12 March at the No. 1 reactor building of Fukushima Daiichi NPP, no triage was performed in the field. The only triage that was performed in the Fukushima accident was at the second explosion on 14 March and the triage was done at a site 4 km away from the plant.

It is recommended that in the event of a radiation disaster, an in-house triage and treatment area should be established on-site where dose rates are reasonably low and there is easy access from the field (Fig. 3.4). The area should have at least an adequate ventilation system, a decontamination room with warm shower, a treatment room, and an area with beds for short stay.

Emergency medical personnel have an important role in on-site response. This is because no medical facilities are available due to the establishment of the restricted area and poor access from outside. The medical team ideally consists of emergency physicians, radiologists, nurses, and radiological technologists. However, the medical team usually comes very late after other responders, and the timing of arrival on the scene depends on radiation levels, access to the restricted area, and available medical resources of the region. The actions of the medical team should be fully incorporated into the joint emergency response in accord with ordinary approaches for MCE (National Center for Injury Prevention and Control 2010).

The medical team approaching to the accident scene should:

- Monitor radiation levels using radiation survey meters and check external dose with personal dosimeter
- Look for evidence of hazardous materials other than radioactive materials

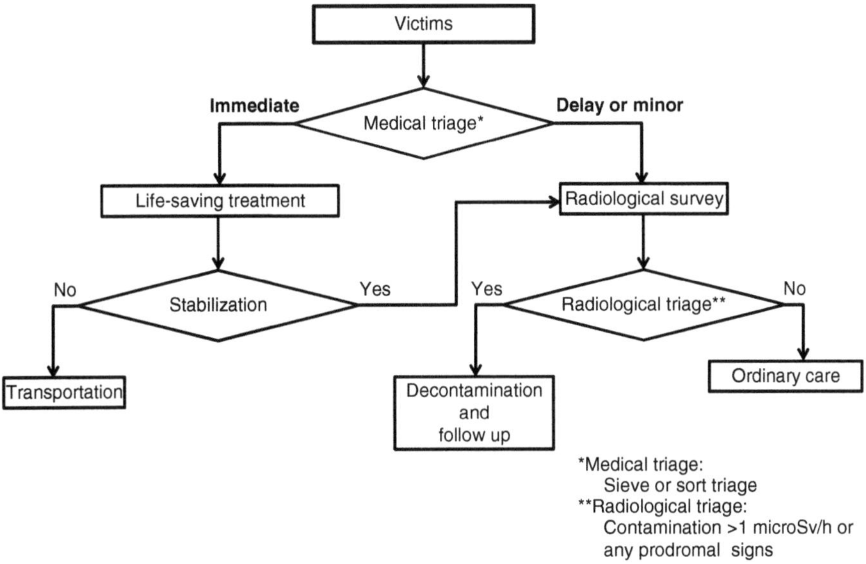

Fig. 3.5 Prehospital triage in a radiation disaster

- Gather information on the exact location, number of casualties, access to the scene, and other emergency services on-site

Well-established command/control and good communication/collaboration/cooperation among related personnel are prerequisites for well-coordinated activities. However, the austere environment, such as exists in a radiation disaster, usually does not allow for this in the conventional manner.

With these limitations, the purpose of medical activities on the scene is to maximize the survival of the majority by triage and by preventing traumatic injuries or illness that would lead to a life-threatening condition, to assess possible contamination, and to perform procedures to control the spread of contamination.

Triage and On-Site Decontamination

Because radiation exposure does not lead to any immediate life-threatening conditions, whereas mechanical injuries or medical problems do, the general emergency medical approach can be applied in the event of a radiation disaster, that is, "Treat life-threatening conditions first!" Therefore, the treatment priority used in prehospital trauma care or cardiovascular life support, and medical triage such as simple triage and rapid treatment (START) triage comes first in MCE (Fig. 3.5) (Benson et al. 1996).

After the patient is stabilized, radiological triage can be started. Radiation levels above background indicate the presence of contamination. In Fukushima, however, difficulties were often encountered in performing accurate radiological evaluation due to high background dose levels. The clinical symptoms such as nausea, vomiting, and diarrhea may constitute the prodromal signs of acute radiation syndrome (Table 3.2) (IAEA 2002b), which requires special attention because early essential actions are required at hospitals.

Table 3.2 Triage categories of radiation injuries according to early symptoms (IAEA 2002b)

	Unlikely	Probable	Severe
Nausea	–	++	+++
Vomiting	–	+	+++
Diarrhea	–	–/+	–/+ to +++
Hyperthermia	–	–	–/+ to +++
Hypotension	–	–	+ to ++
Erythema	–	–	–/+ to ++
CNS dysfunction	–	–	–/+ to ++

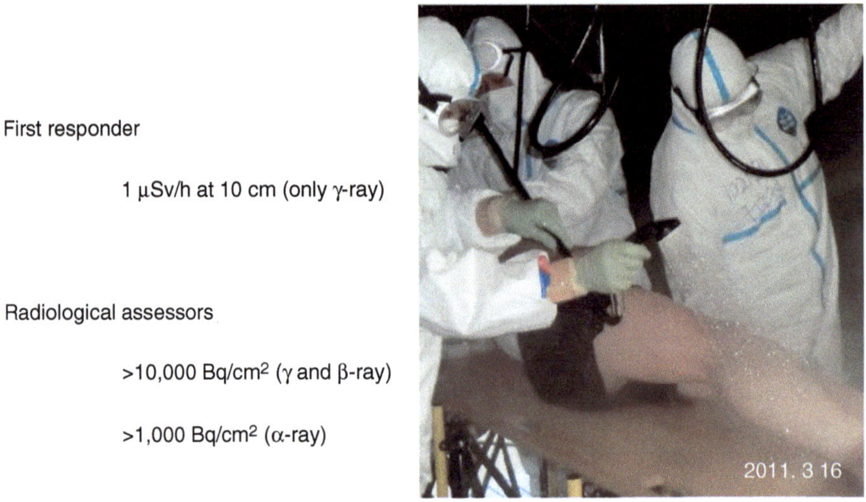

Fig. 3.6 Criteria for on-site decontamination

Once again, there should not be any delay in providing life-saving treatments if it is difficult to perform radiological assessment. If victims are trapped in a vehicle or collapsed building, life-saving maneuvers should be provided during extrication.

Remember that radiation exposure or contamination does not cause immediate signs or symptoms; therefore, if accident victims are unconscious, disoriented, burned, or otherwise in distress, look for causes other than radiation.

Criteria for on-site decontamination of the patient are shown in Fig. 3.6 (IAEA 2006). These criteria indicate the level of skin contamination which could represent a hazard from direct irradiation of the skin, from intake by inadvertent ingestion, or that could indicate that the person has already inhaled or ingested significant amounts of radioactive material. Only one ambient dose rate criterion of 1 μSv/h is provided for use by the first responder. The ambient dose rate criteria were established at levels for strong gamma emitters that can be easily detected under emergency conditions but still correspond to contamination levels more than 100 times below those at which severe deterministic health effects would be expected.

For external contamination, removing outer clothes may get rid of 90 % of radioactive materials attached to the clothes. Wet decontamination using warm water is recommended when feasible. If field decontamination cannot be performed, wrap the contaminated body parts or cover the patient with a sheet or blanket before transportation.

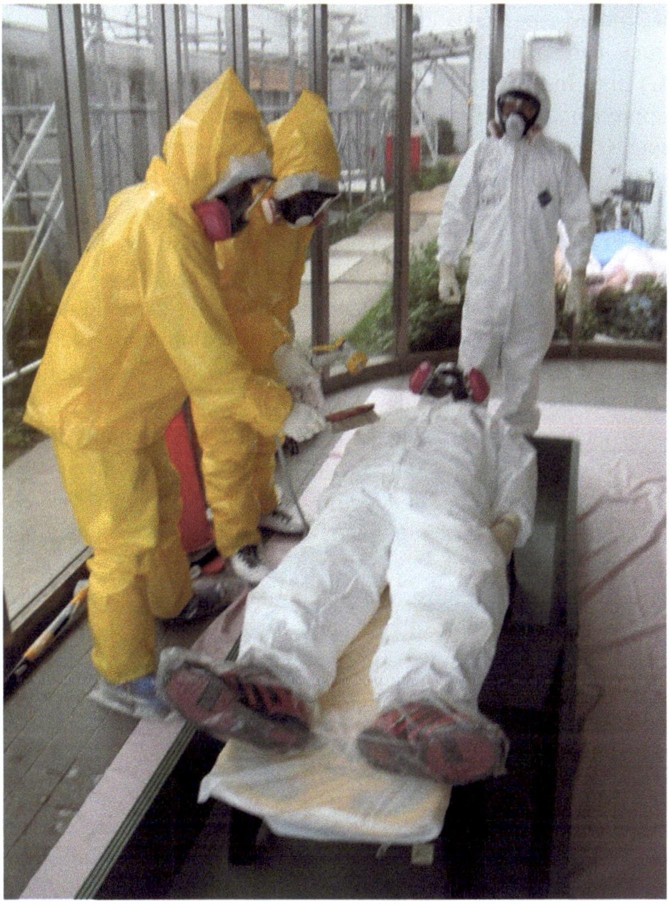

Fig. 3.7 Evaluation of the victim wearing personal protective equipment (PPE) in an in-house triage area

In Fukushima, sufficient water for decontamination was not available due to a massive number of evacuees and disruption of water supply caused by the earthquake. In these circumstances, simply wiping the contaminated skin with wet towels or paper may be recommended.

In cases where absorption of radioactive materials has occurred or is unavoidable, early administration of antidotes or chelates is recommended if the benefits of the medication outweigh the adverse effects of the medication itself (refer to Chap. 2).

Treatment in Prehospital Emergency Settings

Wearing personal protective equipment (PPE) makes it difficult for emergency medical personnel to perform simple activities such as taking vital signs or physical examination. In addition, the victims may be wearing PPE themselves, which interferes with clinical examination such as checking verbal responses, observing respiration or pulse, and performing life-saving maneuvers (Fig. 3.7). Depending on the safety of the scene, i.e., dose rate and any other hazards, it should be determined if provision of initial care on the scene is appropriate.

Example of On-the-Scene Evaluation and Treatment

If the victim is unresponsive, remove the face mask and evaluate level of consciousness (LOC) first. In treating patients with life-threatening conditions, the primary ABCDE approach is usually used (Nolan et al. 2010). The A stands for airway, B for breathing, C for circulation, D for dysfunction of central nervous system, and E for exposure. Any of the airway problems such as disturbed airway due to decreased LOC, airway trauma, or foreign body obstruction should be treated first. In chest trauma, prompt recognition of tension pneumothorax, respiratory failure due to flail chest, and/or pulmonary contusion is essential.

However, examination of the chest is impractical in the field when the victim wears PPE. In this situation, one should focus on breathing only. Only if no respiration or agonal breathing is observed, start cardiopulmonary resuscitation (CPR) if it is possible. Likewise, checking the pulse or capillary refilling is not practical. Observe external bleeding only, and stop active bleeding manually if found.

If the victim is transported to the facility room, ordinary advanced trauma life support or cardiovascular life support may be provided if medical resources are available. Remember, any problems in ABCDE should be managed before radiological survey is started.

In spite of the austere circumstances in a radiation disaster, levels of prehospital emergency care provided in the field should be appropriate to avoid any adverse conditions during transportation.

3.1.3 Establishment of a Command Center

The command center will be positioned in a safe area and as close to the accident site as possible. This location will serve as the center for communication and coordination of all activities to control the emergency and to manage public protection measures. However, in a radiation disaster, the effects of radiation may make it difficult to set up the command center near the site.

In Fukushima, the Fukushima Nuclear Disaster Management Center, where the off-site center was set up to function as a disaster headquarters in nuclear disaster management, was located 4 km from the Fukushima Daiichi NPP. Because of the power and communication failure due to the earthquake, and soaring levels of radiation dose, the center was soon closed (The National Diet of Japan 2012). Although the off-site center were relocated to the Fukushima Prefectural Government office in Fukushima City, practical on-site managements for restoration operations was performed by the command center established at the Japan Football Association's (JFA) National Training Center (known as J-Village), 20 km south from the Fukushima Daiichi NPP (Fig. 3.8). The J-Village served as the headquarters of the Japan Self-Defense Force (JSDF), the fire departments, and Tokyo Electric Power Company (TEPCO) from soon after the accident occurred. The radiation dose rate was within acceptable ranges there, and it had accommodation facilities and a huge football ground suited for a helicopter base. Also, this center was used as a screening site and functioned as a gateway to Fukushima Daiichi NPP of the workers. The J-Village had all the necessary requirements of a command center in a nuclear accident.

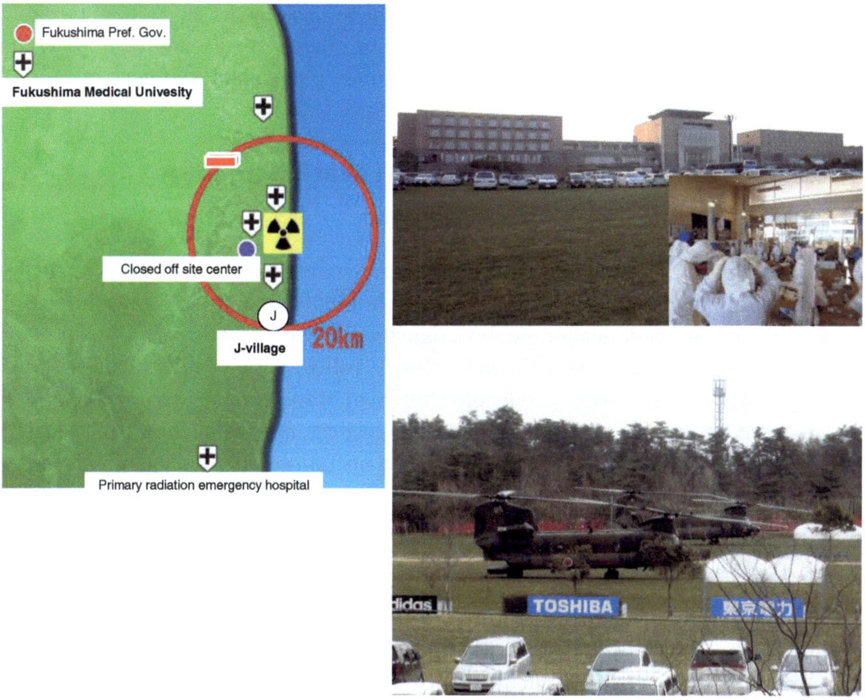

Fig. 3.8 J-Village JFA National Training Center

In preparation, appropriate alternative sites for the command center should be determined in advance, taking factors such as distance, access, and simulated plume dispersion patterns into consideration.

3.1.4 Information on Radiation

Radioactive plume does not spread in a concentric fashion. It spreads while changing its direction quickly due to wind direction, geographic features, and weather conditions. Therefore, information on dose rate and/or prediction of spread pattern of radiation is critical to reduce health risk for all individuals. In Japan, a System for Prediction of Environmental Emergency Dose Information (SPEEDI) had been developed and was expected to play a key role in a severe nuclear accident. However, this sophisticated radiological information system failed due to the strong earthquake in Fukushima (The National Diet of Japan 2012). Instead, mobile monitoring posts had to be introduced to monitor dose rates. However only seven public data spots were available in Fukushima Prefecture, and the results were not provided in a timely fashion (Fukushima Prefectural Government 2011a).

Emergency personnel should monitor radiation dose frequently and protect themselves. For public safety, monitoring of ambient dose rate is required at key spots such as shelters, residential areas, schools, hospitals, and government offices.

Portable monitoring posts should be mobilized to these areas as soon as possible after the accident, and the information should be shared openly among all citizens via any method available such as TV, radio, mobile phone, and Internet.

3.1.5 Development of a Sustainable Local Emergency Medical System

Within a short time after an accident occurs, many individuals will get involved in the restoration operations in the accident facility. In Fukushima, the reestablishment of temporary cooling facilities for the three damaged reactors and the spent fuel pool of the No. 4 reactor building was the first priority, followed by development of stable cooling systems to achieve a stable cold shutdown of the reactors, removal of radioactive debris and rubble, establishment of breakwaters, and installation of a covering container over the No. 1 reactor building. These operations continued until the end of 2011. From 11 March 2011 through 31 March 2012, a total of 19,594 workers were involved in the restoration operations at the Fukushima Daiichi NPP (TEPCO 2012).

3.1.5.1 Emergency Medical Needs of the Workers

In the first month after the accident occurred (March 2011), a total of 67 workers sought emergency medical care including those injured in two hydrogen explosions. Of note is that the majority of them complained of medical problems such as general fatigue and sickness which were unconnected to the levels of radiation dose. Until 30 June 2012, a total of 264 workers had been treated at the site (Fig. 3.9). Three deaths occurred in April, August 2011, and January 2012. Two cases developed cardiac arrest due to acute myocardial infarction. Another case with uncontrolled diabetes died of severe sepsis.

Among emergency care required, trauma accounted for 49.6 % (131 cases). Most of them were observed in the first 5 months after the accident occurred (from 12 March through July 2011). Regarding severity of trauma, only one patient exceeded Injury Severity Score (ISS) of 15. Fortunately, no trauma death was reported. Only six cases were contaminated, all of which occurred in March 2011.

Heat stroke was another concern as the summer season approached. This was because the workers needed to wear PPE. There was an increase in the incidence of heat stroke in May, June, and July. The total number of heat stroke victims was 44, and most of them were treated in Fukushima Daiichi NPP. Only two cases required hospital admission. Repeated advice was provided by TEPCO to all personnel in the Fukushima Daiichi NPP such as wearing cooling jackets under protective suits, taking rest and sufficient fluids regularly, and avoiding any activities from 2 to 4 pm.

3.1.5.2 Irradiation Dose of the Workers

Ninety-six percent of the workers at Fukushima Daiichi NPP were exposed to less than 50 mSv. All of those whose radiation doses were greater than 100 mSv were exposed soon after the accident. A total radiation dose of greater than 200 mSv was

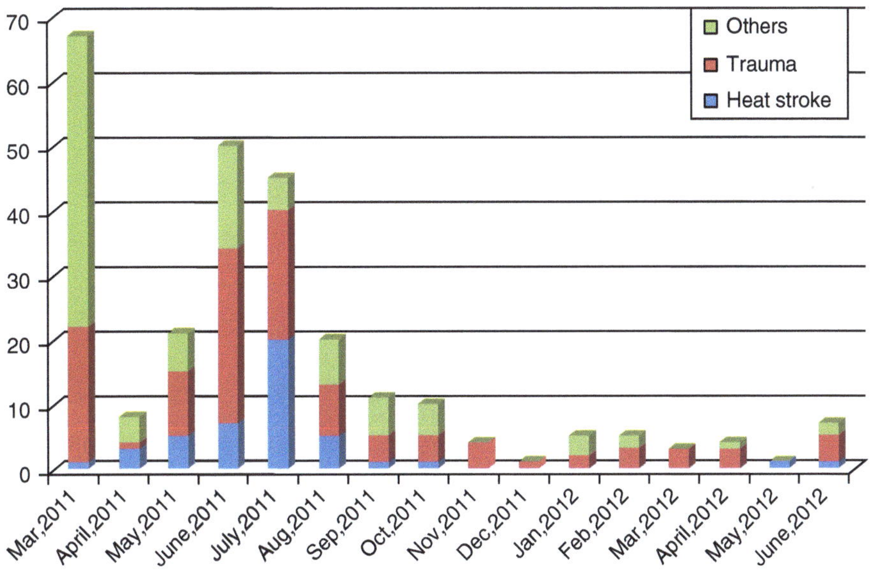

Fig. 3.9 Injuries and illnesses treated at Fukushima Daiichi NPP

Fig. 3.10 Total radiation dose (<100 mSv) of workers who were involved in recovery operations

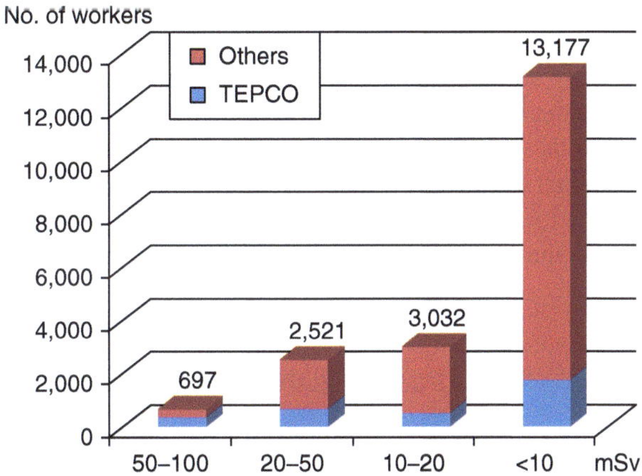

observed in nine workers. Of these, two workers were exposed to greater than 600 mSv with 678 mSv being the highest of all (Figs. 3.10 and 3.11). This worker was engaged in data sampling at No. 3 and 4 reactor building and refueling missions near No. 1 reactor building from 12 March through 15 March. He wore a full face mask with dust filters but without charcoal filters that absorb radioactive iodine. He did not take potassium iodide (The National Diet of Japan 2012).

The workers who had greater than 100 mSv of irradiation dose were regular employees hired by TEPCO. On the other hand, most of those with less than 20 mSv radiation dose were hired by other companies.

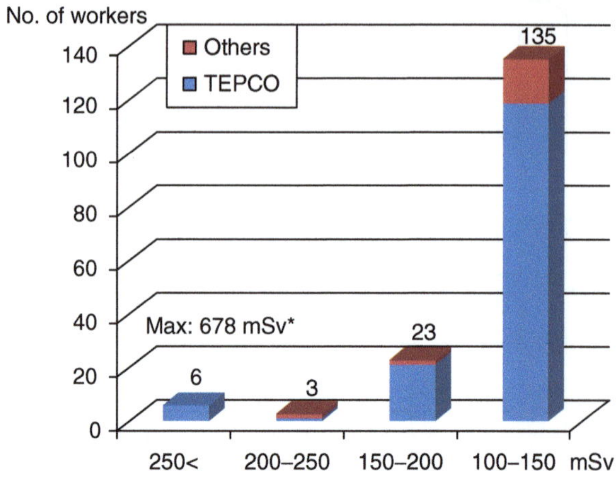

Fig. 3.11 Total radiation dose (>100 mSv) of workers who were involved in recovery operations (11 Mar 2011 to 31 Dec 2011) *Max: 678.08 mSv (Ext. 88.08 mSv, Int. 590 mSv)

Fortunately, no acute radiation syndrome was observed among the affected people in the Fukushima accident.

In a nuclear reactor accident, it usually takes many years to complete decommissioning of the plant. In Fukushima, it took 2 years after the accident occurred before fuel removal from the spent fuel pool commenced. It is likely to take 10 years before the start of fuel debris removal and 30–40 years to complete the decommissioning process (TEPCO 2011). Due to the impact of radiation, medical resources have already diminished. In particular, the number of doctors and nurses has decreased since the beginning of the accident in Fukushima.

In these difficult circumstances, it will become quite challenging to develop a sustainable emergency medical system in the affected region. Strong support from the national government and authorities will be required to develop a system which meets the medical needs in the disaster-stricken area (see Sect. 3.1.8).

3.1.6 Major Public Health Consequences Following Evacuation

The establishment of a restricted zone in a radiation disaster forces large numbers of residents out of the area, where they will stay at temporary shelters or other places for long periods of time. Life conditions in shelters may lead to various types of health issues such as outbreaks of infections, mental stress, and cardiovascular diseases (Math et al. 2008; Ueda et al. 2012; Sun et al. 2013). Sudden changes in lifestyle in unfamiliar places may result in behavioral problems due to poor adaptation to new circumstances. Medical attention will be required from various healthcare disciplines.

In Fukushima Prefecture alone, the number of displaced residents was 86,308 in March 2011, and it reached the peak at 99,205 in June 2011 (Fukushima Prefectural Government 2011b). In addition, the number of residents who voluntarily moved out of Fukushima Prefecture increased from 38,896 in March 2011 to 62,831 in 12 months.

Table 3.3 Medical teams and professions involved in medical activities in the Great East Japan Earthquake from 11 March through 25 May 2011

Teams and healthcare profession	No. of personnel (no. of teams)
DMAT	Approximately 1,500 (approximately 340 teams)
Medical team from national hospitals	471 (92 teams)
Medical team from medical associations	10,354 (2,178 teams)
Pharmacist	1,619
Nurse	1,217
Dentist	220
Physical therapist	60
Public health specialist	6,238 (186 teams)
Mental healthcare team	2,093 (52 teams)

After the Great East Japan Earthquake, more than 460,000 people were displaced to about 2,400 shelters throughout Japan. According to the report on disaster-related death in the Great East Japan Earthquake issued by the Reconstruction Agency of Japan (2012), 2,688 people died at shelters or temporary houses by 31 March 2013. They are called disaster-related death (DRD). DRD is defined as a death caused by deterioration of underlying medical problems due to poor medical access or illnesses arising from poor living environments such as temporary shelters, in a disaster. Ninety percent of DRDs were over 66 years old, and more than one third died within 1 month after the quake. The number of deaths among three Tohoku prefectures was highest in Fukushima (1,383 deaths). The government report indicated that the impacts of the nuclear accident might be the major reason for higher mortality of displaced elderly in Fukushima (Reconstruction Agency of Japan 2012). Another study reported that the impact of the disaster on the excess mortality of institutionalized elderly in Fukushima was most significant in the immediate aftermath because of undesirable living conditions and poor access to medical care (Yasumura et al. 2013). In addition, relocation of these elderly was unavoidable because of the shortage of medical resources in the region, which had a lasting impact on mortality due to continuing changes in nutritional, hygiene, medical, and general care conditions.

Many healthcare professionals headed for the disaster-stricken areas. In less than 2 months after the quake, approximately 24,000 medical personnel were involved in medical activities in Tohoku regions (Table 3.3) (Health and Labor Ministry 2011). However, these medical resources may not have been utilized effectively in Fukushima because concerns over radiation existed; information on radiation and the situation of the vulnerable people was not properly shared nor was sufficient communication among related personnel established during the disaster response (Tanigawa et al. 2011; Tanigawa and Ohjino 2013).

Although the Fukushima accident was combined with a huge earthquake and tsunami, our experiences clearly indicate that the magnitude of the impact of evacuation and displacement on individuals and the society was extremely significant. Proper understanding of radiation by medical personnel as well as citizens cannot be overemphasized. Public healthcare officials and related organization should be well prepared for such an event so that all available medical resources will respond efficiently and effectively to the needs of the region in a radiation disaster.

3.1.7 Summary

The basic goals of prehospital emergency medical response in radiation disaster are the same as other types of disasters. The concept of triage in MCE and treatment priority in the field can be applied likewise. The only difference is the need for protection from the effects of radiation. However, the impacts of radiation on the society including the local emergency medical system are significant. Also, precious medical resources in disasters can be maximally utilized in a radiation disaster. A sustainable emergency medical and public healthcare system which adapt to this specific situation should be developed to cope when any emergency medical needs arise.

3.1.8 Experiences from the Initial Medical Response in Fukushima Accident

In Fukushima, the radiation emergency medical system had been developed within the frame of the national radiation emergency medical system. Six hospitals were designated as the primary radiation emergency medical facility which assumed roles in providing initial treatment and decontamination for victims and one as the secondary radiation emergency hospital (Fig. 3.12).

The effects of radiation forced all residents including medical personnel out of the area, with a 20 km radius from the Fukushima Daiichi NPP (Table 3.4). Three out of the six primary radiation emergency medical hospitals were completely closed because of the evacuation order (Tanigawa et al. 2011). One emergency hospital had lost its function because it was located inside the 30 km radius from the Fukushima Daiichi NPP where indoor sheltering order was issued on 15 March. The closest acute care hospitals were located in Iwaki City, located roughly 44 km to the south of the Fukushima Daiichi NPP. While thousands of workers, fire fighters, and JSDF personnel were vigorously involved in recovery operations, the emergency medical hospitals within the area of a 44 km radius from the Fukushima Daiichi NPP had become virtually unavailable soon after the accident.

As such, the emergency medical system failed when medical resources were in demand (Table 3.5). On 11 March, four workers suffered injuries and two died in the earthquake. On 12 March, the first hydrogen explosion took place at the No. 1 reactor building, and five workers sustained injuries. No field triage was performed. On 14 March, the No. 3 reactor building exploded and 11 workers sustained injuries. In this explosion, an emergency doctor at the off-site center triaged the injured individuals. On the same day, more than 800 patients, who were hospitalized and remained behind at medical or nursing facilities located within a 20 km radius from the plant, were urgently evacuated in 1 day. The information on the patients, i.e., patients' names, conditions, and even the exact number of patients, was not available. They

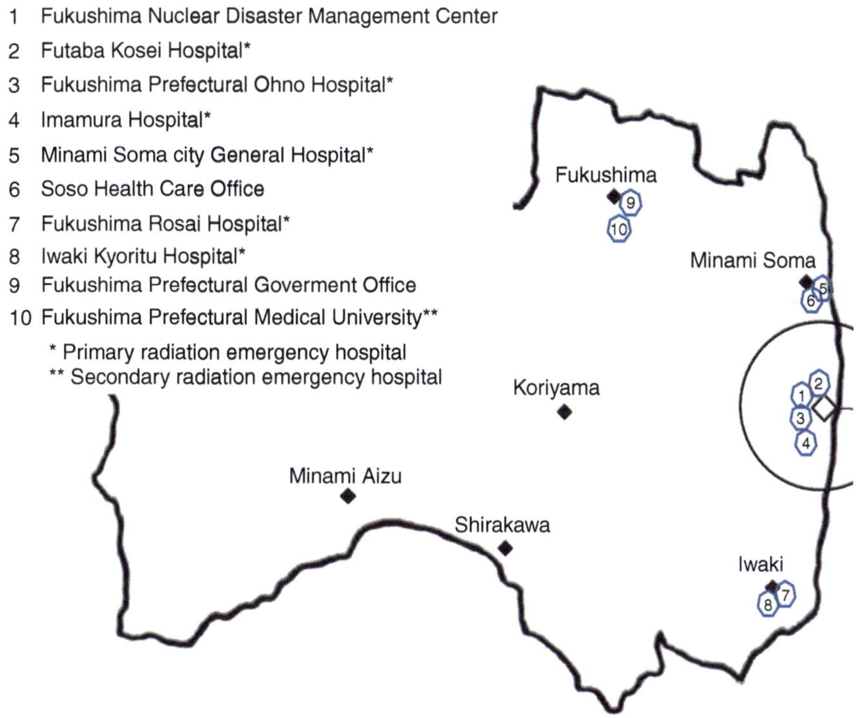

Fig. 3.12 The radiation emergency system in Fukushima before 11 March 2011

Table 3.4 Chronology of the events in Fukushima accident

Date	Time	Events
2011/3/11	14:46	A great earthquake hit eastern Japan, followed by huge tsunamis
	19:03	State of atomic emergency was issued by the national government
	21:23	Evacuation from the 2 km area and indoor sheltering from 2 to 10 km area was ordered
2011/3/12	5:44	Evacuation from the 10 km area was ordered for all residents
	15:36	The first hydrogen explosion occurred at the No. 1 reactor building
		Evacuation of patients in hospitals and facilities was started
	18:25	Evacuation from the 20 km area was ordered
2011/3/13		It was found that approximately 800 patients were left inside the 20 km area
2011/3/14	0:47	Emergency evacuation order was issued for patients in hospitals and facilities inside the 20 km area
	11:01	The second hydrogen explosion occurred at the No. 3 reactor building
2011/3/15	6:00	Severe damage to No. 2 reactor and explosion of No. 4 reactor building occurred
	11:00	Indoor sheltering from 20 to 30 km area was ordered
	15:00	Evacuation of all residents from 20 km area was completed

Table 3.5 Injuries and illnesses required transportation after accident

Date	Injury	Severity	Triage	Contamination	Cause	Methods of transportation	Received hospitals
11 March	Fracture of lower extremities	Severe	Not done	No	Earthquake	Ambulance	Hospital in Koriyama
	Laceration on head	Minor	Not done	No	Earthquake	Facility vehicle	Ono Hospital (designated hospital)
12 March	Subarachnoid hemorrhage	Severe	Not done	No		Facility vehicle	Hospital in Koriyama
	Open fracture of the femur	Moderate	Not done	No	Explosion	Facility vehicle	Initially treated at a clinic (non-designated facility) and transferred to a hospital in Koriyama
	Contusion of lower extremity	Minor	Not done	No	Explosion	Facility vehicle	Treated at a clinic (non-designated facility)
	Contusion of upper extremity	Minor	Not done	No	Explosion	Facility vehicle	Treated at a clinic (non-designated facility)
	Contusion	Minor	Not done	No	Explosion	Facility vehicle	Treated at a clinic (non-designated facility)
	Severe tinnitus	Minor	Not done	No	Explosion	Facility vehicle	Treated at a clinic (non-designated facility)
	Headache, nausea	Minor	Not done	No		Facility vehicle	Treated at off-site center (OFC)

14 March	Fracture of clavicle, scapula	Moderate	Done at OFC	Yes	Explosion	Ambulance	Fukushima Medical University (FMU)
	Dislocation of shoulder joint	Moderate	Done at OFC	No	Explosion	SDF vehicle	Treated at OFC
	Laceration of thigh	Moderate	Done at OFC	No	Explosion	SDF helicopter	National Institute of Radiological Sciences (NIRS)
	Contusion on thigh	Minor	Done at OFC	No	Explosion	SDF vehicle	Treated at OFC
	Laceration of foot	Moderate	Not done	Yes	Explosion	Facility vehicle	Initially treated at Fukushima No. 2 NPP, transferred to FMU on 15 March
	Laceration of foot	Moderate	Not done	Yes	Explosion	Facility vehicle	Initially treated at Fukushima No. 2 NPP, transferred to FMU on 15 March
	Contusion on chest	Minor	Not done	Yes	Explosion	Facility vehicle	Initially treated at Fukushima No. 2 NPP, transferred to FMU on 16 March
	Contusion on chest, upper extremity	Minor	Not done	No	Explosion	Facility vehicle	Initially treated at Fukushima No. 2 NPP, transferred to FMU on 16 March
	Contusion on foot	Minor	Not done	No	Explosion	Facility vehicle	Treated at Fukushima No. 2 NPP
	Contusion on elbow	Minor	Not done	No	Explosion	Facility vehicle	Treated at Fukushima No. 2 NPP
	Contusion on upper extremities	Minor	Not done	No	Explosion	Facility vehicle	Treated at Fukushima No. 2 NPP

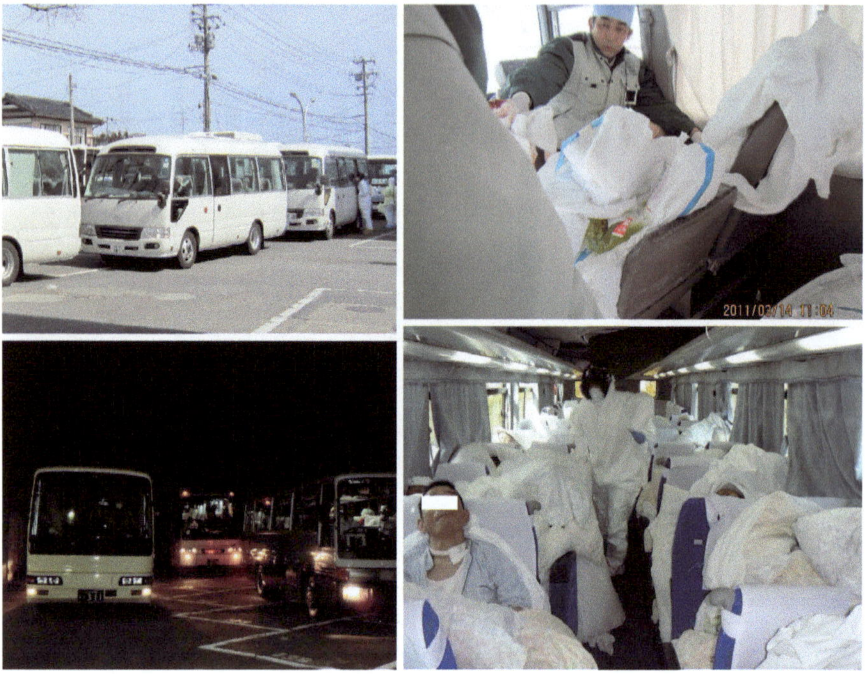

Fig. 3.13 Evacuation of inpatients. Patients were evacuated by chartered buses (*upper left and bottom right*) and police vehicles (*bottom left*). A patient fell down from the seat during evacuation and required an emergency treatment for head injury (*upper, right*)

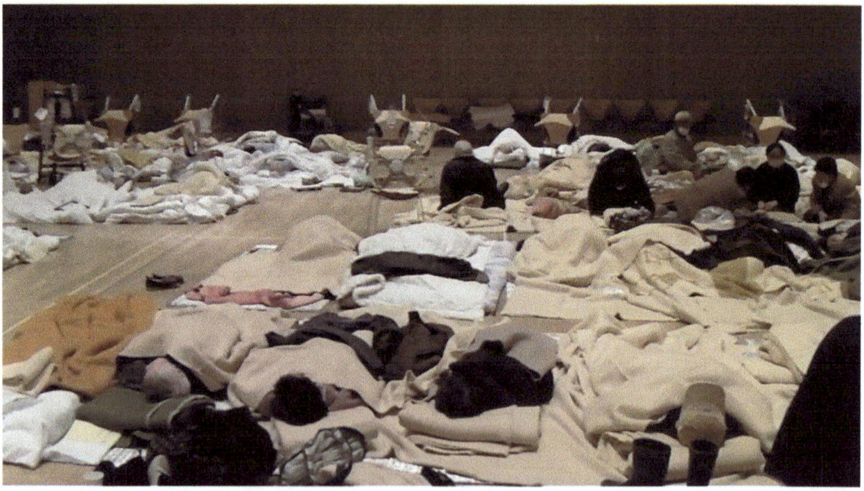

Fig. 3.14 Evacuated patients housed in a shelter in Fukushima

were transported by buses or police vehicles for a relatively long time; however, no medical personnel were in attendance and no medical care was provided during or after evacuation (Figs. 3.13 and 3.14). Unfortunately, 60 elderly patients died in this evacuation. Hypothermia, deterioration of underlying medical problems, and dehydration were suspected as the causes of death (Tanigawa et al. 2012).

On 15 March 2011, the national government ordered the evacuation of all hospitalized patients and elderly in care facilities in the indoor sheltering zone, 20–30 km radius from the plant, because of the shortage of medical supplies and commodities in this area. At this time, the Disaster Medical Assistance Team (DMAT) headquarters at the Ministry of Health, Labour and Welfare planned and arranged evacuation of more than 400 patients with support of DMATs (Kondo et al. 2011). DMAT is a specially trained medical team for disasters, consisting of one doctor, two nurses, and a logistic person (Kondo et al. 2009). Many ambulances and JSDF vehicles were mobilized at this time, and DMATs were engaged in triage of the patients at collection sites and in providing medical care before and during evacuation (Fig. 3.1). Although it took 4 days to complete, the evacuation was done safely without any casualty.

Since soon after the accident occurred, thousands of individuals had been involved in the restoration operations every day. There was an urgent need for reinstallation of cooling systems for the reactors and nuclear fuels. On 24 March, two workers were exposed to high levels of contaminated water on their feet in the basement of the No. 3 reactor building. Fortunately, they did not sustain any trauma or acute radiation syndrome.

No medical doctors were available in the Fukushima Daiichi NPP for the first week after the accident. Unfortunately, one worker developed full cardiac arrest at the Fukushima Daiichi NPP on 17 March and was transported by a facility vehicle to a hospital located 44 km south from the Fukushima Daiichi NPP. Thereafter, part-time occupational physicians started to see the facility workers at the Central Building of the Fukushima Daiichi NPP (Kinugasa 2012). Meanwhile, efforts had been made to reestablish the emergency medical response system with support from the local government, the national government, various organizations, and medical societies.

At the J-Village, located 20 km south of Fukushima Daiichi NPP, there was a medical facility which served as a sport medicine facility for football players. This facility was later renovated as a primary radiation emergency medicine facility (Figs. 3.8 and 3.15). In case of MCE, the first triage for the victims would be performed on-site and the second triage and emergency care would be provided at the J-Village (Morimura et al. 2012). However, marked delay was still unavoidable because of the distance of J-Village from the Fukushima Daiichi NPP.

As the restoration activities increased, the Japanese government decided to set up a 24-h emergency care facility at the Fukushima Daiichi NPP. This is so-called 5/6 ER because it was established by renovating the first floor of the Unit 5/6 reactor management building, which was located 600 m north of the Unit 1 reactor building (Figs. 3.16, 3.17, and 3.18). The dose rates around the Unit 5/6 reactor service building ranged from 10 to 15 μSv/h, which were relatively low compared to other areas in the Fukushima Daiichi NPP. However, there were areas of high dose rates (100–200 μSv/h) on the route from the 5/6 ER to the Central Management Building or the gate of the Fukushima Daiichi NPP. In addition, it was located in the center of the restricted area where only authorized personnel and vehicles were allowed to enter.

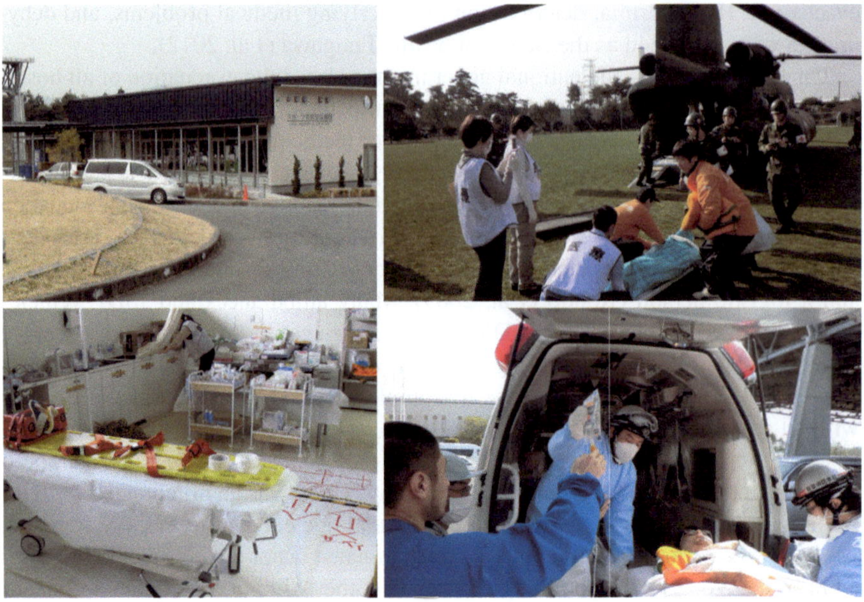

Fig. 3.15 The medical facility in J-Village (*left*). Patients were triaged and treated here before being transferred to hospitals

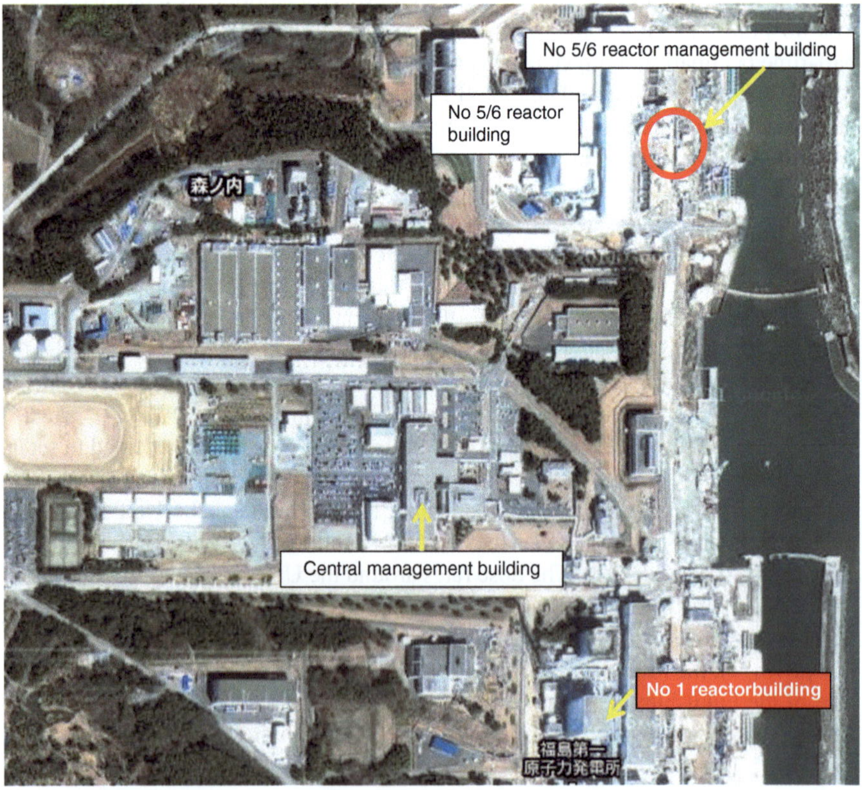

Fig. 3.16 Fukushima Daiichi NPP and Unit No 5/6 reactor building https://maps.google.co.jp/

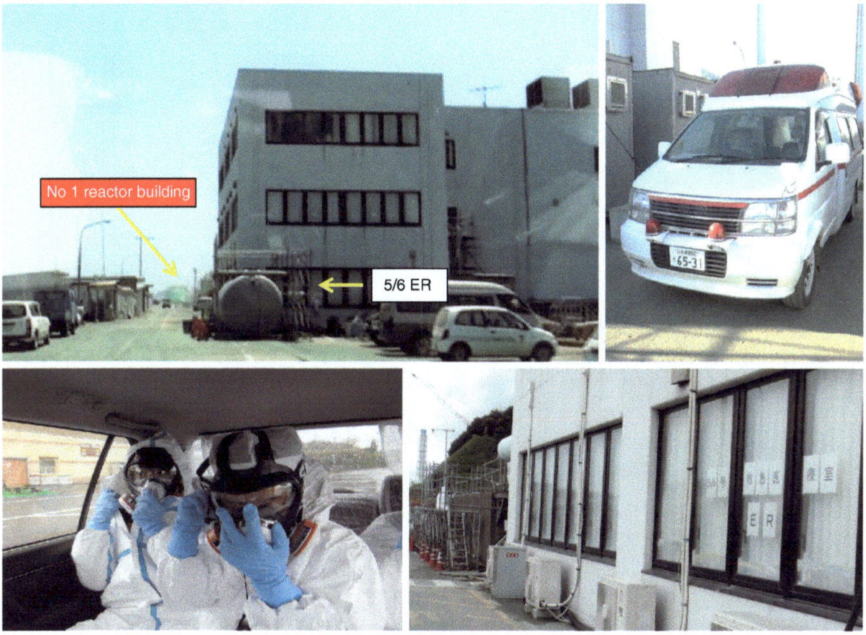

Fig. 3.17 Unit No 5/6 reactor Management building (*upper, left*) and 5/6 ER (*bottom, right*). Full PPE was required to reach 5/6 ER (*bottom, left*). *Upper right* is ambulance for emergency dispatch and transportation

Furthermore, the road conditions surrounding the Fukushima Daiichi NPP remained disrupted. Therefore, no immediate access to referral hospitals was available.

In order to provide appropriate emergency medical treatments in this specific environment, emergency physicians, nurses, and radiological technicians experienced with radiological emergencies were recruited from all over Japan. They took 48-h shifts in order to limit radiation exposure to themselves. Because no immediate medical assistance was available within the area of the 44 km radius from the Fukushima Daiichi NPP, we had developed a telemetric system which transmitted high-resolution live images to affiliated facilities (Fukushima Medical University, Hiroshima University, National Institute of Radiological Sciences) so that the medical team of the 5/6 ER was able to obtain medical information and advice necessary for various types of medical emergencies.

In order to coordinate all efforts for the emergency medical system as well as provide adequate occupational environment for workers in the plant, we had set up the Emergency Medical System Network (Fig. 3.19). This network consists of TEPCO, the national government, University of Occupational and Environmental Health, National University hospitals, Occupational Disease hospitals, National Institute of Radiological Sciences, and the Japan Society of Acute Medicine. Hiroshima University has been organizing this network (Fig. 3.19). One of the biggest challenges for us was the recruitment of medical

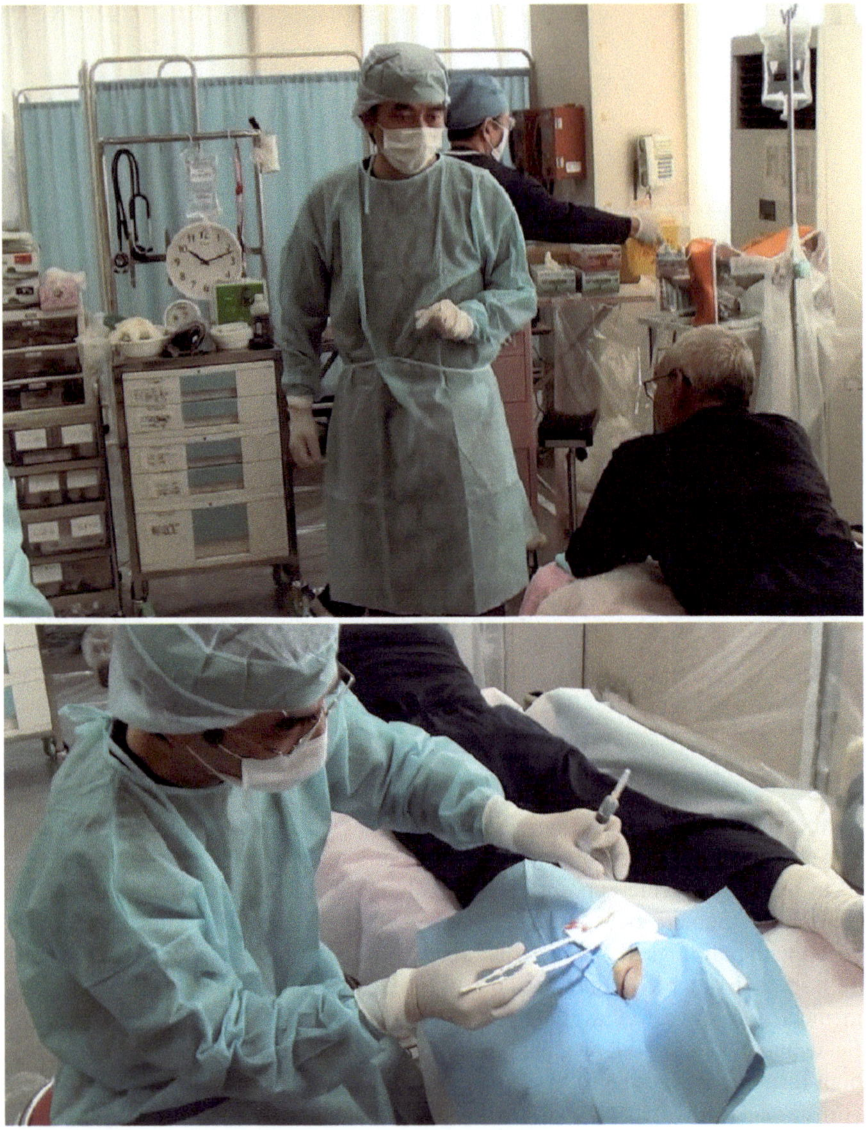

Fig. 3.18 Patient care in 5/6 ER with limited medical resources

staff that were willing to serve in these difficult circumstances. We needed physicians and nurses who had competence in emergency and disaster medicine but who in addition had a good understanding of radiation. We had detailed discussion on the occupational environment and preventive medicine particularly in the warm and cold seasons. Also follow-up of workers with chronic illnesses and mental health needs were discussed with the help of University of Occupational and Environmental Health.

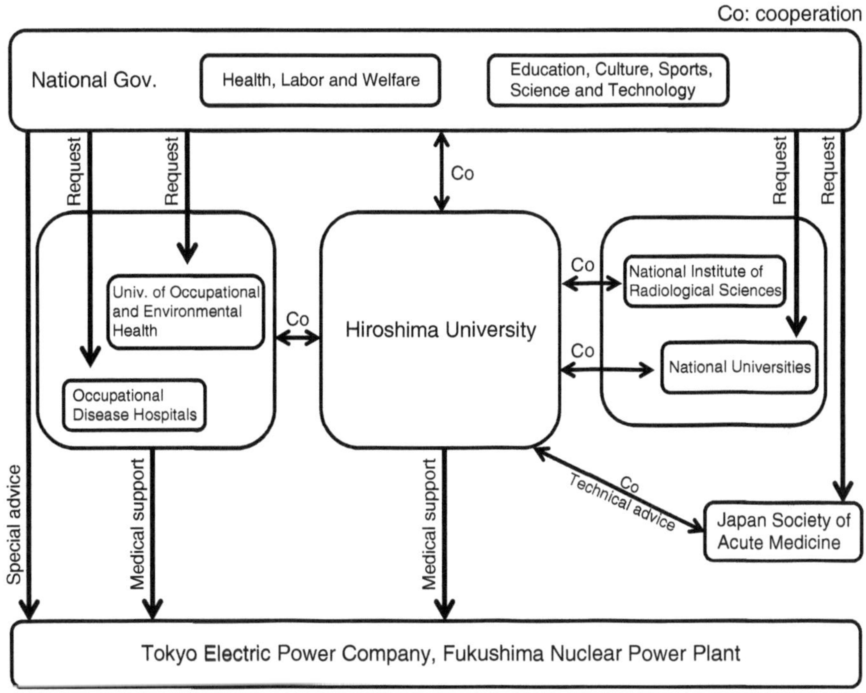

Fig. 3.19 TEPCO Fukushima nuclear power plant emergency medical system network

3.1.8.1 Disaster Response of Medical Professionals and Societies in the Great East Japan Earthquake

In disasters, the modern structure of medicine, that is, specialty-based medicine, may not be applicable to the needs in the region due to marked imbalance between medical needs and resources (shortage of doctors, equipment, and facilities). Medical care in disasters, therefore, is not specialty based but medical needs based. In the acute phase of disasters, triage and life-saving treatment for trauma or life-threatening illnesses are put as first priority. This is the major reason for the development of Disaster Medical Assistance Teams (DMATs) in Japan (Fig. 3.20) (Kondo et al. 2009). Doctors in DMAT are required to finish a special DMAT training program in addition to the Japanese Advanced Trauma Evaluation and Care (JATEC) course or similar training courses (Trauma Training Course Developing Committee of JAST and JAAM 2002). Basically, their background specialties are related to acute care for injured victims, i.e., emergency medicine, anesthesiology, general surgery, neurosurgery, and orthopedic surgery.

On the other hand, general medical needs for displaced people in shelters or temporary houses include care for common illnesses, underlying medical problems, mental health, dental care, maternal care, rehabilitation, and prevention of communicable diseases. These fall under the area of family medicine, primary care medicine, and public health and were managed by medical teams from governmental or

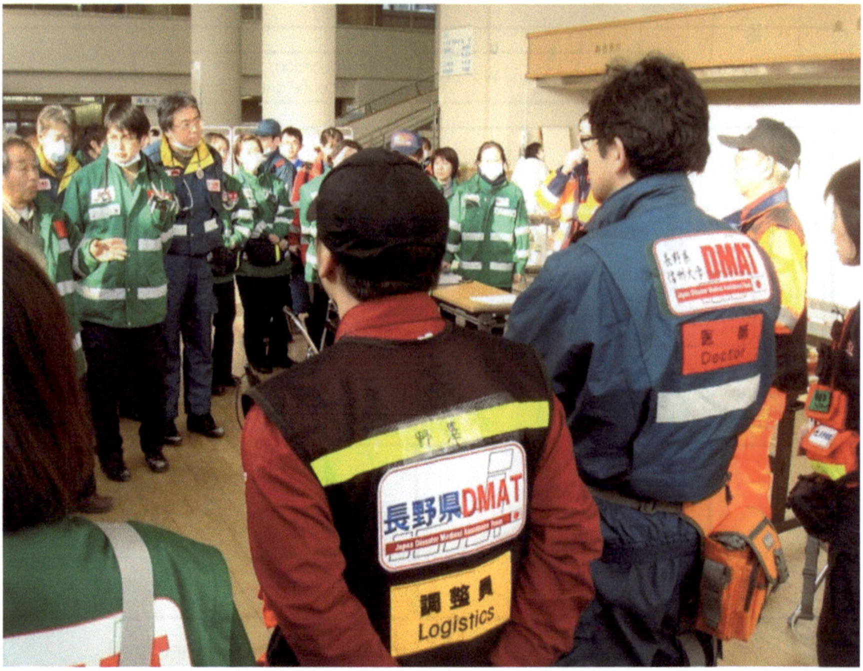

Fig. 3.20 DMATs from all over Japan gathered at designated disaster hospitals in the Tohoku region (13 March 2011)

nongovernmental organizations such as the national hospitals (Health and Labor Ministry 2011), the Japan Medical Association (JMAT) (Ishii 2011), and the Red Cross hospitals. The doctors of these medical teams represent a wide variety of medical specialties. The knowledge and skills required for general care are fundamentals of medical training and, therefore, are supposed to be obtained during residency programs in Japan, yet general care is still currently underdeveloped. This is one of the major reasons for which the national government has been trying to strengthen general medicine since the Great East Japan Earthquake.

Unfortunately in Fukushima, many doctors including emergency physicians were initially unwilling to serve in medical activities related to the Fukushima accident (Tanigawa et al. 2011; Tanigawa and Ohjino 2013). In this difficult situation, the Japan Association for Acute Medicine (JAAM) decided to support Fukushima as a professional medical society of emergency and disaster medicine soon after the accident. They sent core members of the society to the off-site center of the nuclear disaster management headquarters in Fukushima City and to the

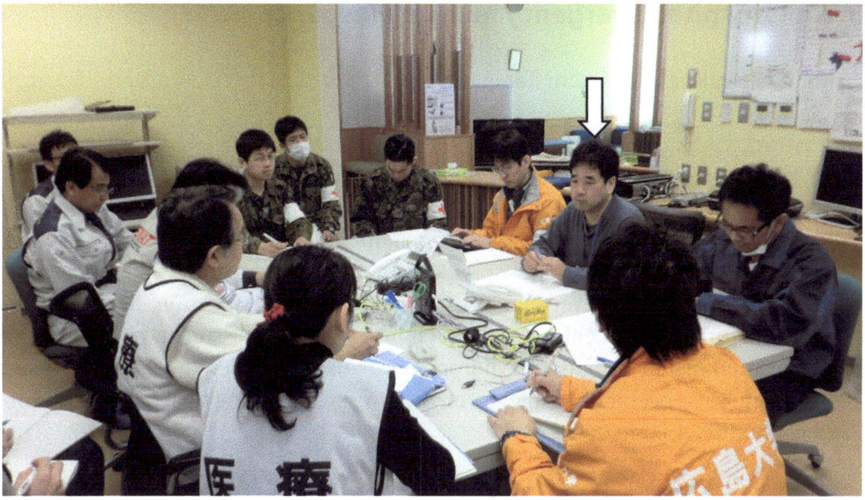

Fig. 3.21 A member from the Japan Association for Acute Medicine (JAAM) (indicated by *arrow*) coordinated medical activities at the J-Village with the Japan Self-Defense Force (JSDF) personnel, specialists from Hiroshima University, National Institute of Radiological Sciences (NIRS), and Tokyo Electric Power Company (TEPCO) on 13 April 2011

J-Village, to coordinate medical activities and provide advice as disaster medicine specialists (Morimura et al. 2012) (Fig. 3.21). For their commitment, the JAAM was awarded a special letter of appreciation from the national government in 2013 (JAAM 2013).

Acknowledgments: The author would like to acknowledge Dr Penelope Engel-Hills for her editorial assistance and helpful comments.

3.2 Hospital Emergency Medical Response

Arifumi Hasegawa and Koichi Tanigawa

Abstract
In a radiation disaster, the loss of important functions of the preexisting medical response system due to the impact of radiation is expected. This chapter outlines the planning and general considerations in the hospital emergency medical response. Various aspects of hospital emergency response are explained including preparation, patient reception, triage, radiological evaluation, decontamination, and further treatment for radiation injuries. Dose assessment, local radiation injury, and acute radiation syndrome are also considered in this chapter. Experiences of hospital emergency medical response during the Fukushima accident are discussed in detail.

3.2.1 Introduction

In a radiation disaster, one should expect a substantial functional loss of the preexisting medical system due to the impact of radiation on the region. Not only hospitals and chronic care facilities in an evacuation zone but also others outside the zone may be affected. In Fukushima, severe dysfunction of the radiation emergency medical system in the region was encountered soon after the accident (Tanigawa et al. 2011).

Planning should be developed taking these circumstances into consideration, and should there be a radiation event, the emergency medical response should be made with maximal support from not only the local government but also the national government, authorities, and medical societies/associations.

3.2.2 Planning

A protocol for hospital response in radiation disaster should be integrated in general disaster planning including all hazard protocol for chemical, biological, radiological, nuclear, and explosives (CBRNE) events (Valentin and International Commission on Radiological Protection 2005).

Victims in a radiation disaster may not necessarily be transferred to the designated hospitals. Therefore, the hospital emergency department should have a plan and a protocol for the delivery of prompt and appropriate medical care to the victims while minimizing the effects of radiation on the victims, healthcare team, their equipment, and the facility. To prepare for the worst case scenario, an

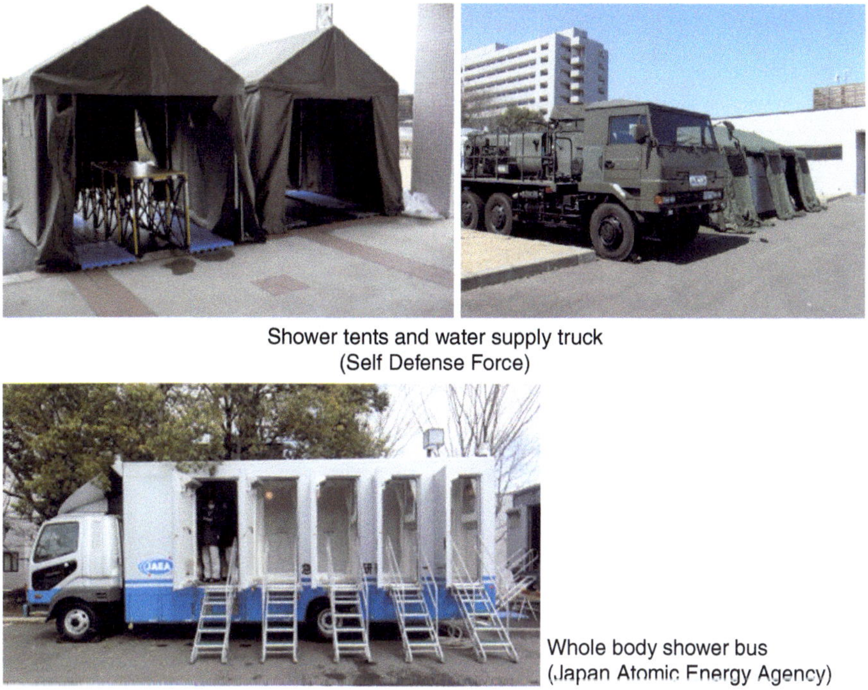

Fig. 3.22 Decontamination facilities at Fukushima Medical University (FMU)

evacuation plan of the hospital itself should be included if the hospital is located close to a nuclear facility.

In the early phase of a radiation disaster, the hospital emergency department may be overloaded with patients. At the same time, the hospital may suffer from functional damage, due to the departure of medical personnel who leave because of fear of radiation. This is what happened in Fukushima.

The number and severity of victims with radiation injuries and/or contamination determines the initial medical resources required: how many medical institutions, staff members, transport vehicles, equipment, supplies, etc. that should be mobilized. Also, plans must be available for transfer of excess victims to other hospitals. Medical resources from other regions across the entire nation should be mobilized and utilized effectively to support the hospitals in the disaster-stricken region.

In Fukushima, the Japan Self-Defense Force (JSDF) and other organizations deployed the decontamination corps and mobile facilities to Fukushima Medical University (FMU) (Fig. 3.22). The doctors, nurses, radiology technicians, and radiation specialists from other institutions headed for FMU to support the existing medical activities at FMU.

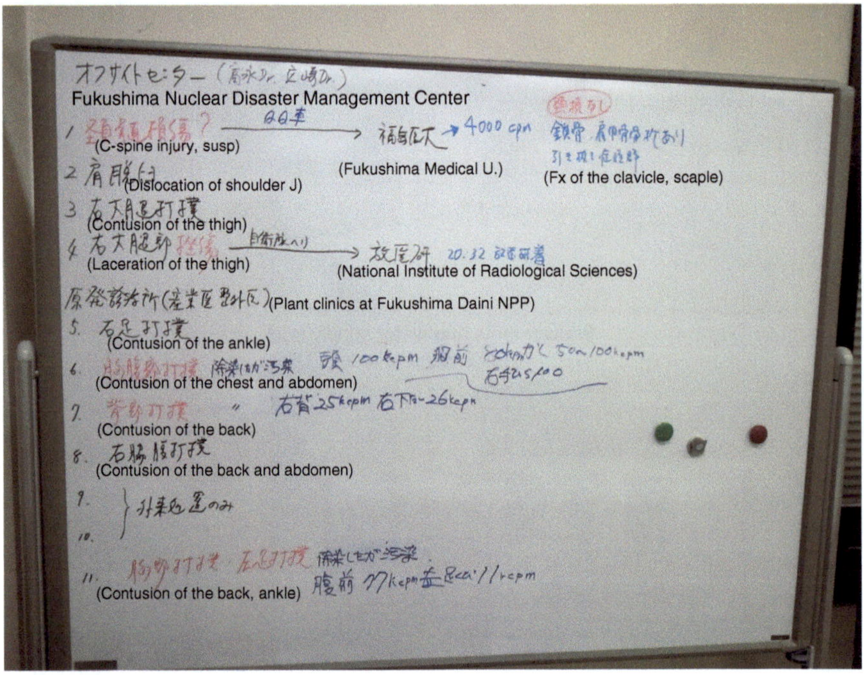

Fig. 3.23 Clinical data of workers injured during the hydrogen explosion on 14 March. Only limited information on victims available from the site

3.2.3 General Considerations of Hospital Response

In a radiation disaster, proper initial care may not be provided at the site of the accident. Information on the number of victims, medical status, and radiological status such as contamination and exposure may not be available or may be confusing (Fig. 3.23). In these situations, hospital staff should be prepared to receive multiple casualties with contaminated trauma and radiation injuries.

The principle in the initial medical response is basically the same as ordinary mass casualty events (MCEs) (see Chap. 3). Medical triage should come first, followed by life-saving treatments and followed by radiological evaluation. Any victim of a radiation accident must be considered as contaminated until proven otherwise.

3.2.4 Hospital Emergency Response

In these difficult situations, a basic course of action in the hospital emergency department includes (International Atomic Energy Agency [IAEA] 2002c):

1. Preparation
2. Patient reception
3. Triage and life-saving treatment

4. Radiological evaluation
5. Decontamination
6. Further radiological evaluation and treatment for radiation injuries

3.2.4.1 Preparation

3.2.4.1.1 Before Patients' Arrival

After being notified of the arrival of victims in a radiation accident involving contamination, the emergency response team, including radiological specialists, should prepare for patient reception.

Special preparation measures include protection of the medical staff, hospital facility, and equipment while preventing the spread of contamination outside a designated area. The medical team should be prepared to receive any severely injured, heavily overexposed victims that have a combination of injuries and contamination with radioactive materials.

When the hospital receives a call that radiation accident victims are to be admitted, a planned course of action should be followed. The individual receiving the call should get as much information as possible, including:

1. Number of accident victims
2. Each victim's medical status
3. Whether victims have been monitored for contamination
4. Radiological status of victims (whether exposed or contaminated)
5. Type of radioactive material, its activity/concentration, and whether it is detected on the skin surface of the victim or on their clothes
6. Estimated time of arrival at hospital

Information on victims should be shared and the planned course of action of each member should be decided at a briefing before the arrival of the victims (Fig. 3.24).

Hospitals should also be prepared for the uncertain situation when there is a lack of accurate information. In this case, hospital staff have to prepare for CBRNE events.

3.2.4.1.2 Preparation of a Radiation Emergency Area (REA)

An REA consists of a decontamination and treatment room. The purpose of the REA is to protect both facilities and personnel from the spreading radionuclides that contaminated the victims.

When selecting the site for an REA, the following should be taken into consideration:

- REA should have an outside entrance or easy access.
- REA should be away from the main traffic flow.

A triage area should be established at the entrance, prior to the decontamination and treatment rooms of the REA (Fig. 3.25).

Non-contaminated patients are admitted to the usual treatment area, while contaminated patients must be admitted to the specially prepared decontamination area first.

Ventilation in the REA should be turned off if it is part of the general ventilation system. It is most appropriate to equip the REA with an isolated ventilation system.

Life support and other essential medical equipment and supplies should be available immediately and ready for use. All nonessential equipment in the room is removed or covered (Fig. 3.26).

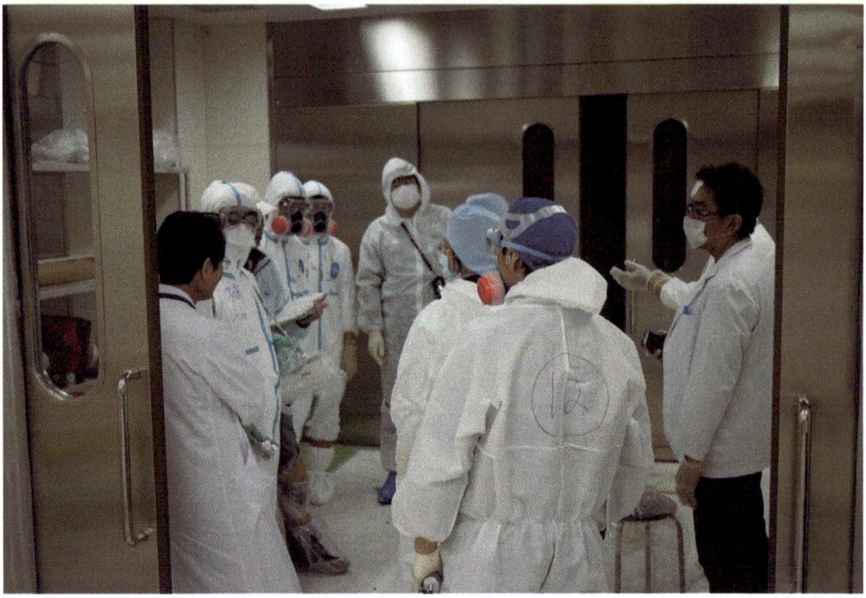

Fig. 3.24 Briefing before arrival of the victims at FMU

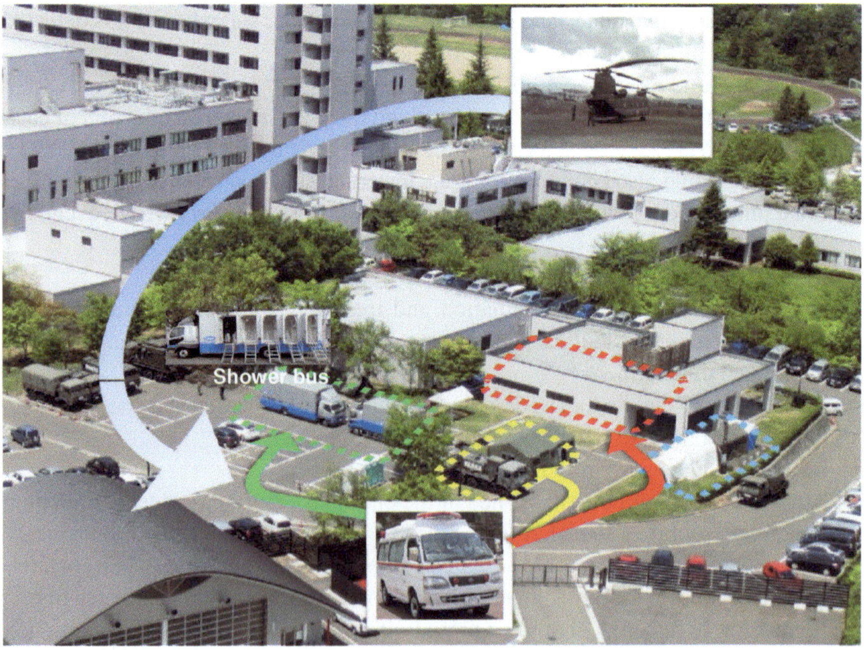

Fig. 3.25 Triage site and patient flow (*red arrow*: urgent, *yellow*: delay, *green*: minor). *Blue area* is a decontamination tent; *red area* is the radiation emergency area (REA) (FMU)

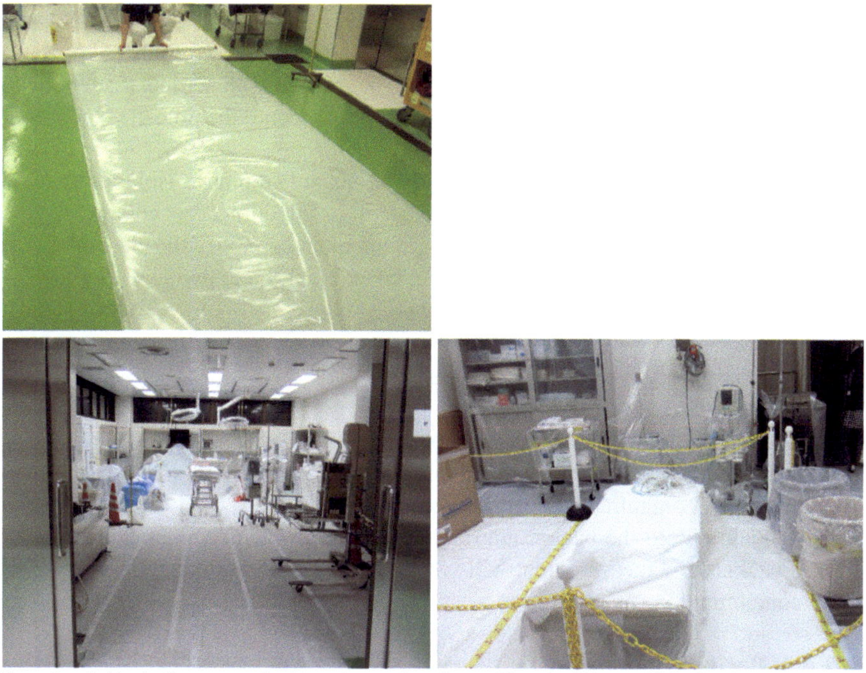

Use rolls of wide plastic or paper sheet to make a path from the ambulance entrance to the decontamination room. Ordinary cloth sheets or square absorbent pads can be used if paper is unavailable. The floor of the decontamination room or treatment area should be similarly covered.

A control line should be established at the entrance to the decontamination room. By marking clearly using a wide strip of tape on the floor at the entrance, the contaminated side should be differentiated from the non-contaminated side.

Fig. 3.26 Preparation of a radiation emergency area (REA) at FMU

3.2.4.1.3 Preparation of Medical Staff

Once alerted, the radiation safety personnel must provide each member of the radiation emergency hospital team with personal dosimeters and must prepare survey meters to conduct radiological evaluations on all victims in order to evaluate for contamination.

While the facility is being prepared, members of the radiation emergency response teams should be dressed in surgical attire: scrub suit, gown, mask (covering both nose and mouth), cap, and gloves. Two pairs of gloves should be worn. The first pair of gloves should be under the arm cuff and secured by tape. The second pair of gloves should be easily removable and replaced if they become contaminated. Waterproof shoe covers should also be used. Other staff should wear protective gear and personal protection as necessary.

The purpose of protective clothing is to keep bare skin and personal clothing of contaminants. This protective clothing is effective in stopping alpha and beta particles but not gamma rays. Lead aprons, however, such as those used in the radiology department, are not recommended since they are heavy to use and give a false sense of security. They will not stop most gamma rays that have higher energy than X-rays.

Remember, the victim of exposure without contamination poses no radiological hazard to anyone else. However, there is a risk to the victim. If exposure is known or suspected, a CBC (count of blood cells) should be ordered with particular attention to determining the absolute lymphocyte count. Be sure to record the time the blood sample is taken.

Procedures in handling of contaminated victims are similar to isolation precautions and to the protocol for patients with contagious infection. This will prevent the spread of contaminants to the hospital environment and simplify the cleanup.

It is reasonable to assume that the route taken from the ambulance to the REA can become contaminated.

3.2.4.1.4 Preparation of Survey Meters

Prior to patient arrival:

- Check if radiation monitors function properly.
- Cover the probe of the radiation monitor with a sheet of cling film and secure with tape. A contaminated cover can easily be removed and replaced.
- Check and record the background radiation level in the decontamination room. The background measurement will serve as a reference point in assessing levels of contamination.

3.2.4.2 Patient Reception

The medical team receives the radiation accident victim at the ambulance or other transporting vehicle. Ambulance personnel should stay with the vehicle until they and their vehicle are monitored and released by radiation safety personnel (Fig. 3.27).

3.2.4.3 Triage and Life-Saving Treatment

The critically injured patient should be taken immediately into the prepared REA. Primary ABCDE approach for medical evaluation can be used in a radiation accident (Nolan et al. 2010): immediate assessment of the victim's airway, breathing, and circulation should be made and any necessary life-saving measures performed. In case of MCE, medical triage should be performed first. Life-saving interventions should be carried out before decontamination.

3.2.4.4 Radiological Evaluation

Immediate treatment for life-threatening conditions should be done prior to the radiological evaluation (Fig. 3.28). When placing an intravenous line, blood sampling should be done for blood cell counts and biodosimetry. Nasal swabs must be taken to check with a gross beta, gamma, and alpha counter whether the patient inhaled radioactive aerosols or alpha particles. If radioactivity above the normal background level is detected, the nasal swab and the positive skin smears should be taken for gamma spectrometry to identify the isotope composition responsible for contamination.

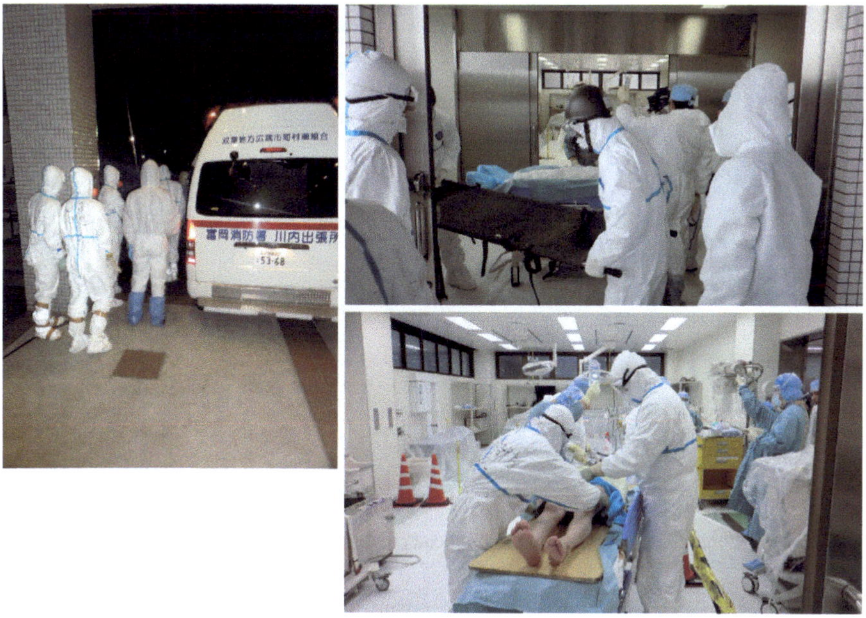

Fig. 3.27 Patient reception and radiation emergency area (REA) at FMU. Arrival at FMU (*left*). Transport of patient from ambulance to REA (*upper right*). Medical evaluation of patient (*bottom right*)

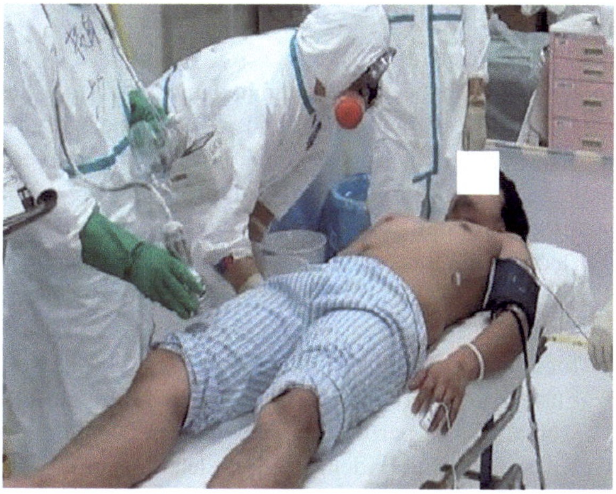

Fig. 3.28 Radiological evaluation of a patient at Fukushima Medical University. This patient was physically stable; a radiological survey was performed while a brief case history was being taken

If the victim's condition allows, an initial, brief radiation survey should be performed to determine as soon as possible if the victim is contaminated. If a radiation survey meter reading indicates the possibility of contamination, a more thorough survey will be performed in the decontamination room.

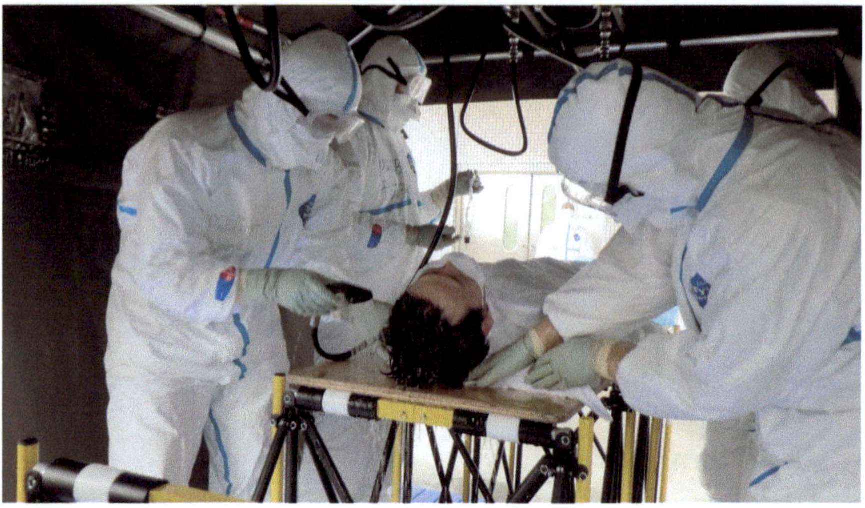

Fig. 3.29 Decontamination of a worker with head contamination (FMU)

If the victim's contaminated clothing has not been removed yet, remove it in or near the ambulance or in the decontamination room and place it in a plastic bag. Personal belongings and items used in patient care should be bagged, labeled (name, date, hour), and saved for examination by the radiation safety personnel.

3.2.4.5 Decontamination

Intact skin can be decontaminated using warm water with soap or orange oil (Fig. 3.29). Contaminated wounds can be repeatedly washed with saline or, if necessary, excised. During decontamination procedure, pay close attention to the patient status to avoid any delay in providing life-saving measures if their medical status deteriorates.

Decontamination endpoint is reached when:

1. The contamination is low enough to no longer be a significant hazard, i.e., twice the background level. The patient may leave the REA following a careful survey for contamination with radioactive materials at exit.
2. Further decontamination procedures would cause more damage to the skin or wound. This is particularly true in case of contaminated wounds of hands or face, where further debridement might lead to significant tissue deficit.
3. In MCE, decontamination procedure cannot be completed if numbers of victims overwhelm available medical resources. If decontamination is not completed, cover the contaminated part of the body (Fig. 3.30). Contaminated areas in the stratum corneum layer of the skin will desquamate with epidermis in normal metabolism.

3.2.4.6 Further Radiological Evaluation and Treatment

Following the radiological triage, the patient with suspected radiation exposure of unknown severity should be transferred to a designated medical institution capable

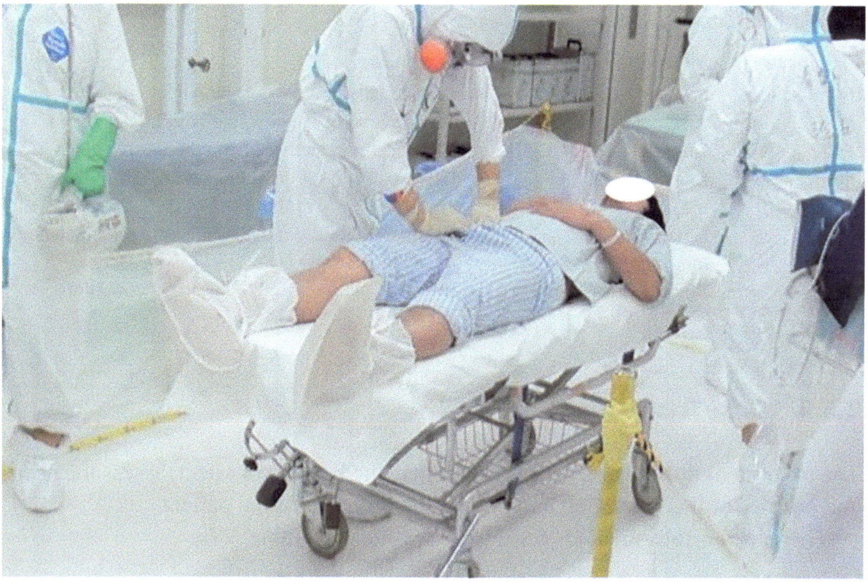

Fig. 3.30 Partial body decontamination. Area not decontaminated was covered by a sheet

Table 3.6 Types of radiation injuries, severities, and treatments

Type of exposure	Health consequence	Treatment at a hospital
Localized exposure, more often to hands	Localized erythema with or without signs of development of blisters, ulcers, and necrosis	Desirable in a general hospital: Clinical observation and treatment Specialist advice is necessary in severe cases
Total or partial body exposure with minimal and delayed clinical sign	No clinical manifestation for 3 h or more following exposure Not life threatening! Minimal hematological changes	Clinical observation, symptomatic treatment, and sequential hematological investigations are necessary in a general hospital
Total or partial body exposure with early prodromal symptoms	Acute radiation syndrome of moderate to severe degree dependent on dose	Treatment required in specialized hospital Early full blood count and human leukocyte antigen (HLA) typing are essential
Total or partial body exposure with severe injury	Possible severe combined injuries, life threatening	Treat life-threatening conditions Early transfer to a specialized center is necessary

of identifying radiation-induced effects. This assessment, called the extended triage, will inform further evaluation and treatment including dose assessment and decorporation/decontamination treatment as necessary (Table 3.6) (IAEA 2002d).

Table 3.7 Method of dose assessment

Classification	Methods	Examples
Biological	Somatic symptom	Prodromal symptoms of the ARS
	CBC	Time course of the absolute lymphocyte count
	Chromosomal analysis	Chromosomal analysis from the lymphocytes
Physical	Radiation source measurement	Density of the skin contamination, dermal absorption ratio at the depth of 0.07 mm
	Environmental measurement	Calculate with the radiation quantity and distance from the source
	Physical measurement	Bioassay methods and the external counting devices

3.2.5 Dose Assessment

The purpose of dose assessment is to estimate the biological effect, assess the needs and priority of the treatment, and predict the outcome of the patient.

There are various methods for dose assessment as Table 3.7

3.2.6 Local Radiation Injury (LRI)

Patients who may have received a high dose to a limited area of the body require continuing care of the localized radiation injury. Patients with LRI (hand, feet, thigh, etc.) will experience signs and symptoms of thermal burns except for marked delay in the onset of clinical changes, from several days to weeks after exposure.

Basic clinical symptoms of LRI by acute exposure of gamma radiation of high-dose rate are shown in Table 3.8 (IAEA 2005).

Deep ulceration and necrosis may be able to be treated with the dosimetry-guided resection and autologous mesenchymal stem cell therapy (Lataillade et al. 2007).

3.2.7 Acute Radiation Syndrome (ARS)

Acute radiation syndrome (ARS) is a combination of clinical syndromes occurring in stages during a period of hours to weeks after a large portion of a person's body is exposed to a high dose of radiation. The timing and extent of the injury manifestations depend upon the type, rate, and dose of radiation received. The percentage of the body that is injured, the dose homogeneity, and the intrinsic radiosensitivity of the exposed individual also influence manifestations. Different ranges of whole-body doses produce different manifestations of injury.

Table 3.8 Basic clinical symptoms of local radiation injury (LRI)

	Severity grade and corresponding dose of exposure, Gy			
Phase of LRI	Grade I (mild) 8–12 Gy	Grade II (moderate) >12–30 Gy	Grade III (severe) 30–50 Gy	Grade IV (very severe) >50 Gy
Initial reaction (initial erythema)	Lasts for several hours, can be absent	Lasts from several hours to 2–3 days	Lasts from 2 to 4–6 days. Expressed in all exposed individuals	Expressed in all exposed individuals until the manifestation period.
Latent period	Up to 15–20 days	Up to 10–15 days after exposure	Up to 7–14 days after exposure	N/A
Manifestation period	Secondary erythema	Secondary erythema, edema, blistering	Secondary erythema, edema, pain syndrome, blistering, erosions, initial radiation ulceration, pus infection	Edema, pain syndrome, local hemorrhages, necrosis
Conclusion of LRI development	Dry desquamation by 25–30 days	Moist desquamation, with development of new epithelium under rejected layer by the end of 1–2 months	Development and healing of ulcers is delayed and takes months. Deep ulcers do not heal without surgical treatment (skin grafting)	Processes of injury delineation and rejection are delayed. At 3–6 weeks there is development of gangrene with general intoxication and sepsis. Only timely and radical operation can save life
Delayed effects (consequences)	Skin dryness, pigmentation	Atrophy of skin, subcutaneous layer, and muscles is possible; late radiation ulceration	Scarring and epithelium defects; deep trophic, degenerative, and sclerotic changes; initial necrosis	Effects of amputation, ulcer relapses, contractures

The three main ranges that produce the most characteristic manifestations are referred to as the hematological, gastrointestinal, and neurovascular syndromes. High-dose injuries to smaller percentages of the body produce local injury effects but may not cause ARS.

Table 3.9 Clinical symptoms and prognosis of acute radiation syndrome (ARS)

Symptoms	Treatment
No nausea, vomiting, or diarrhea Lymphocyte count above 1,000 mm–^{3} at 48 h Probably no life-threatening injury	Observe periodically for any change in clinical status
Nausea, mild vomiting, conjunctiva redness, and erythema Lymphocyte count between 700 and 1,000 mm–^{3} at 48 h	Probably injury with mild grade of severity; plan for therapy
Pronounced nausea and vomiting; possible diarrhea, conjunctiva redness, and erythema Lymphocyte count between 400 and 700 mm–^{3} at 48 h	Probably life-threatening injury; plan for maximum therapy in specialized hospital
Prompt severe vomiting and bloody diarrhea, erythema, and hypotension	High probability of lethal outcome
Lymphocyte count between 100 and 400 mm–^{3} at 48 h	Provide with maximum therapy in specialized hospital
Loss of consciousness Prompt severe vomiting and bloody diarrhea, erythema, and hypotension Lymphocyte count below 100 mm–^{3} at 48 h	Low probability of survival. Provide with supportive therapy

3.2.7.1 Clinical Symptoms of ARS

An accident involving tens or hundreds of individuals exposed, or suspected of exposure, would cause great difficulties, especially in hospitalization. Thus, planning is very important and should be adapted to the medical system contemplated for catastrophic event situations. This chain of sorting and care becomes crucial, especially when both medical resources and facilities are limited. Early estimation of prognosis would be necessary in a mass casualty scenario (Jackson et al. 2005; Dainiak et al. 2011a).

The early clinical symptoms serve as the basis of sorting persons exposed to radiation and deciding on proper medical care at an individual level. The most important prodromal early clinical signs are nausea, vomiting, and diarrhea.

However, estimation of the degree of radiation damage and exposure is often difficult; therefore, sequential diagnosis and reassessment are mandatory throughout the patient's clinical course. Prodromal symptoms begin within hours of exposure. The prodromal gastrointestinal symptoms generally do not last longer than 24–48 h after exposure, but a vague weakness may persist for an undetermined length of time. The time of onset, severity, and duration of these symptoms are dose and dose-rate dependent and should be used in conjunction with early biological parameters, such as granulocyte and lymphocyte levels, to determine the presence and severity of ARS (Table 3.9) (IAEA 2005).

3.2.7.2 Treatments of ARS

Decision of treatment for acute radiation syndrome (ARS) should be based on the symptoms, evolution of medical status, and laboratory results. The World Health

Table 3.10 Summary of recommendations for treating 100–200 hospitalized patients with whole-body exposure to ionizing radiation

Syndrome	Recommendation	Strength of recommendation
Gastrointestinal	Administer fluoroquinolone or similar antibiotic 2–4 days after radiation exposure	Weak (B-1b)
	Provide bowel decontamination and parenteral antibiotics when indicated, if resources permit	Weak (C-1b)
	Administer a serotonin-receptor antagonist prophylactically when suspected exposure is >2 Gy	Strong (A-1a)
	Administer loperamide pro re nata for control of diarrhea	Weak (B-1b)
	Provide nutritional support through enteral route	Weak (B-1b)
Cutaneous	Administer topical class II–III steroids, topical antibiotics, and topical antihistamines to radiation burns, ulcers, or blisters	Strong (A-1a)
	Administer systemic steroids for radiation burns, ulcers, or necrosis in the absence of a specific indication for systemic steroid use	Strong against (D-2a)
	Surgically excise and graft radiation ulcers or localized necrosis with intractable pain	Strong (B-1a)
Neurovascular	Provide supportive care with a serotonin receptor antagonist, mannitol, furosemide, and analgesics	Strong (A-1a)
Critical care	Administer fluid and electrolyte replacement therapy and sedatives when significant burns, hypovolemia, and/or shock occur	Strong (A-1a)
	Administer mechanical ventilation with a lung-protective strategy for acute respiratory failure	Strong (A-1a)
	Administer SOD or SDD to decontaminate the digestive tract	Weak (B-1b)
	Maintain average blood glucose of 140–180 mg/dL for majority of critical care patients	Weak (B-1b)
	Administer H2 blocker or proton pump inhibitor	Weak (B-1b)

Strength of recommendation was determined by assignment of quality of the evidence (A-high, B-moderate, C-low, or D-very Low) and strong (1a) or weak (1b) recommendation in favor of the practice. Strong (2a) recommendation is against the practice

Organization convened a panel of experts to rank the evidence for medical countermeasures for management of ARS and hematopoietic syndrome (HS) in a hypothetical scenario involving the hospitalization of 100–200 victims (Dainiak et al. 2011a, b). Although high-quality studies of therapeutic interventions in humans are not available, the panel compiled recommendations for treatments for ARS and HS (Tables 3.10 and 3.11). Further research is needed to identify new therapeutic approaches and countermeasures for radiation injuries.

The concept of ARS has recently shifted from the single organ failure, dependent on the exposed dose, to the multiorgan dysfunction syndrome including bone

Table 3.11 Summary of recommendations for treating hematopoietic syndrome in hospitalized patients with whole-body exposure to ionizing radiation

Recommendation	Strength of recommendation
Administer G-CSF or GM-CSF when ANC < 0.500×10^9 cells/L	Strong (B-1a)
Administer ESAs when prolonged anemia is present to avoid need for red blood cell infusion	Weak (C-1b)
Administer hematopoietic stem cells after failure of 2–3 week of cytokine treatment to induce recovery from marrow aplasia in absence of nonhematopoietic organ failure	Weak (D-1b)

Strength of recommendation was determined by assignment of quality of the evidence (A-high, B-moderate, C-low, or D-very low) and strong (1a) or weak (1b) recommendation in favor of the practice
ANC absolute neutrophil count, *ESA* erythropoiesis-stimulating agents, *G-SF* granulocyte colony-stimulating factor, *GM-CSF* granulocyte macrophage colony-stimulating factor

marrow, skin, lung, gastrointestinal tract, and the central nervous system (Jackson et al. 2005). Therefore, the therapy should be provided by a multidisciplinary team consisting of the critical care specialists, general internists, hematologists, oncologists, plastic surgeons, dermatologists, vascular surgeons, psychiatrists, and consultants in other medical specialties. Cooperation among these specialists is needed to optimize patient outcomes.

3.2.8 Summary

In a radiation disaster, planning for hospital response should be developed assuming a decreased function of the regional medical system due to the impact of radiation. Mobilization of resources and interhospital cooperation and coordination will play a key role in saving the lives of those who are severely injured and in treating radiation injuries as well. Treatment modalities, in accord with the recent recommendations, should be taken into consideration for ARS and HS, although stronger evidence for treatment of radiation injuries requires further time and research.

3.2.9 Experiences from Fukushima Accident

The radiation emergency medical system in a region should be developed within the frame of the national radiation emergency medical system. Before the Fukushima accident, 77 hospitals were designated as the radiation emergency facility which was to play the key roles in case of a radiation emergency in Japan. However, our system had not been prepared for a radiation disaster. After the Fukushima Daiichi nuclear power plant (NPP) accident, four radiation emergency medical hospitals were closed due to evacuation; two hospitals lost effective function partially as a result of doctors and nurses leaving due to concerns over radiation risk in Fukushima.

Eventually, the Fukushima Medical University (FMU) Hospital was the only one left to cope with the emergency response including radiation accidents.

While we were involved with emergency care for patients with trauma, hypothermia, drowning, and other conditions caused by the earthquake and tsunami, the situation at the Fukushima NPP was deteriorating. The first explosion at the plant took place on 12 March, and the evacuation order was issued. On 13 March, many evacuated patients were urgently transported to FMU. This was the first severe nuclear power plant accident that occurred in Japan. Information was so scarce, and we had no idea what was happening at the site, what the effects of radiation would be, and what would happen next at the power plant and to us. Anxiety, concern, and uncertainty overwhelmed us. We were at a loss (Hasegawa 2012).

On the next day, 14 March, the second explosion took place and injured workers were transported to FMU before we were able to prepare for such events. Although we had hospital response plans before the accident, we were not adequately prepared. Many hospital staff were facing with the crisis.

Of great help at this critical moment were the medical assistant teams from Hiroshima University, Nagasaki University, National Institute for Radiological Sciences, and Nuclear Safety Research Association (Fig. 3.31). They gave us lectures on basic knowledge on the effects of radiation and countermeasures in a severe reactor accident (Fig. 3.32). In addition, they helped us prepare for the events and provided initial treatment for contaminated victims. Their presence was quite encouraging not only technically but also mentally and emotionally. From that moment, we were better prepared for the events including MCE.

Acknowledgments The authors would like to acknowledge Dr. Penelope Engel-Hills for her helpful comments and editorial assistance.

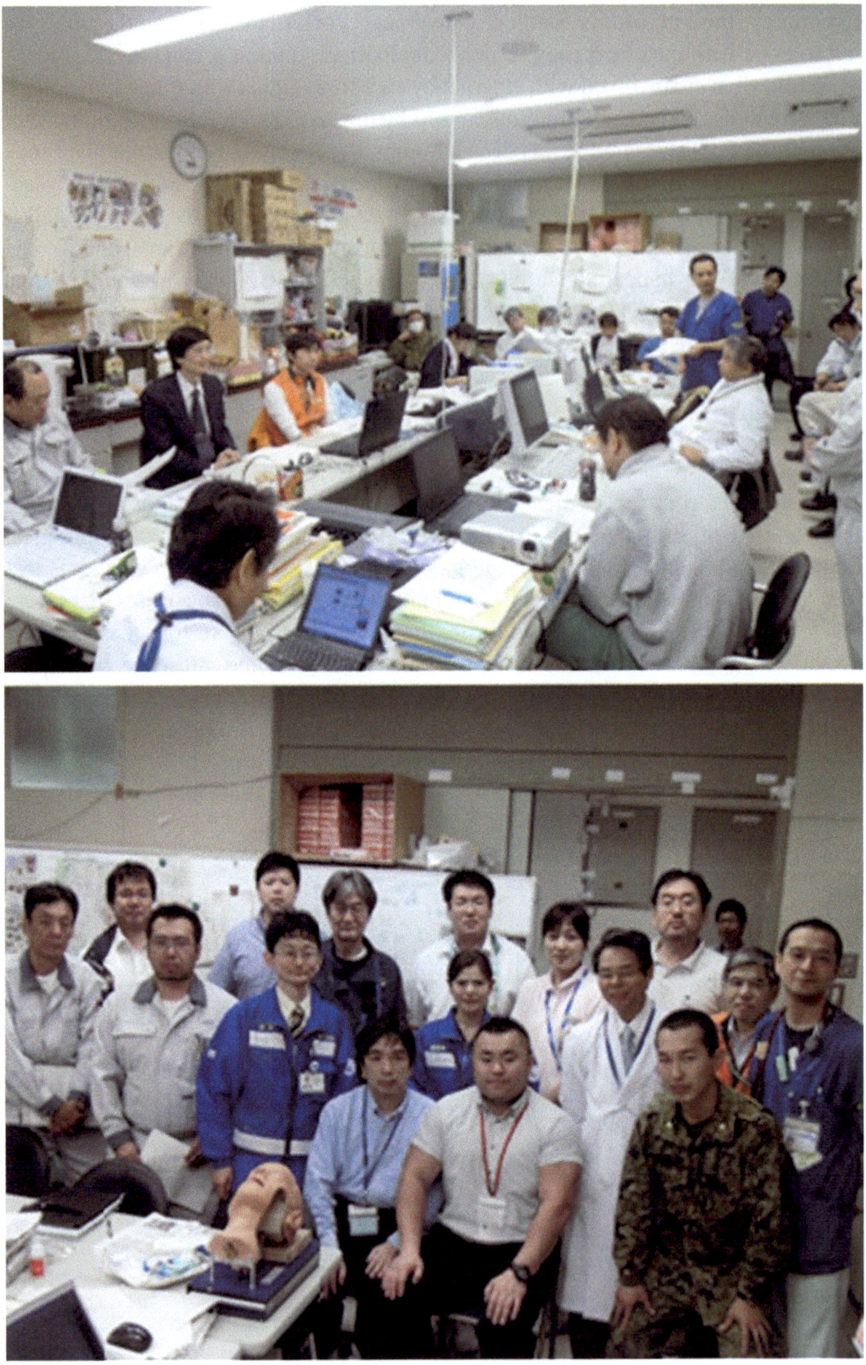

Fig. 3.31 FMU hospital staff and medical assistant teams from other institutions (at FMU)

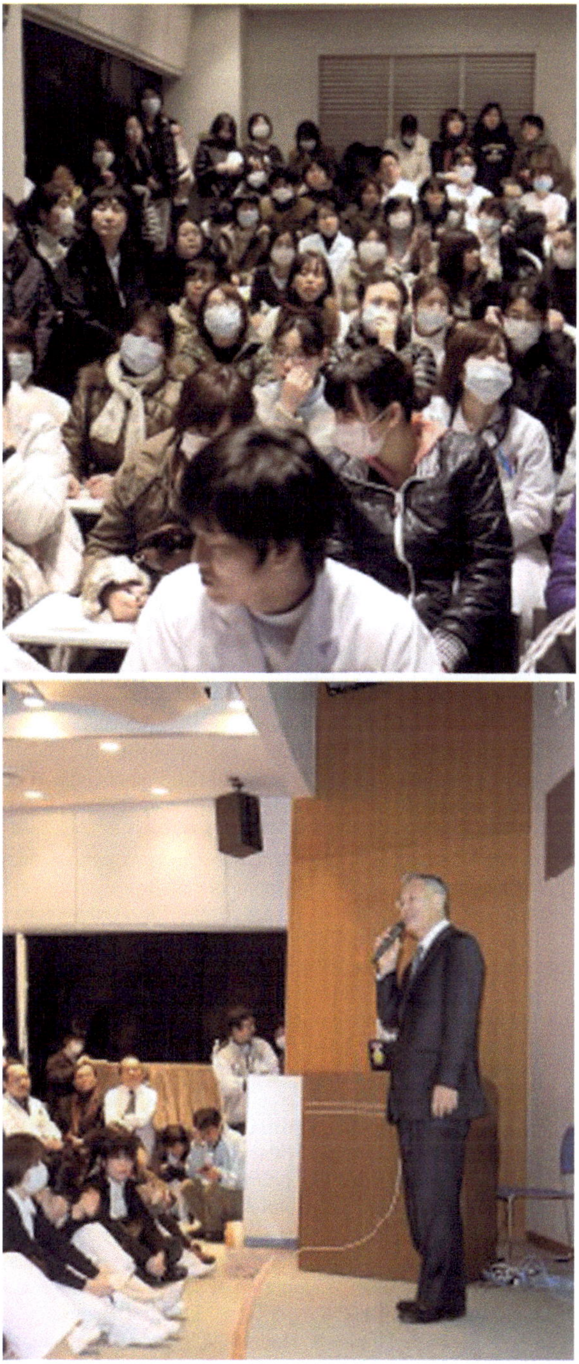

Fig. 3.32 Briefing to anxious hospital staff by Professor Yamashita from Nagasaki University soon after the accident

References

Benson M, Koenig KL, Schultz CH (1996) Disaster triage: START, then SAVE – a new method of dynamic triage for victims of a catastrophic earthquake. Prehosp Disaster Med 11(2):117–124

Dainiak N, Gent RN, Carr Z et al (2011a) Literature review and global consensus on management of acute radiation syndrome affecting nonhematopoietic organ systems. Disaster Med Public Health Prep 5(3):183–201. doi:10.1001/dmp.2011.73

Dainiak N, Gent RN, Carr Z et al (2011b) First global consensus for evidence-based management of the hematopoietic syndrome resulting from exposure to ionizing radiation. Disaster Med Public Health Prep 5(3):202–212. doi:10.1001/dmp.2011.68

Fukushima Prefectural Government (2011a) Interim report of radiation dose rates in 7 sites in Fukushima prefecture. http://www.pref.fukushima.jp/j/7houbu0311-0331.pdf. Accessed 1 April 2011 (in Japanese)

Fukushima Prefectural Government (2011b) Current status of displaced residents in Fukushima. http://wwwcms.pref.fukushima.jp/. Accessed 1 Aug 2011 (in Japanese)

Hasegawa A (2012) Activities of radiation medical group in Fukushima Medical University. Mook Iryokagaku 5:59–68 (in Japanese)

Health and Labor Ministry (2011) Report on damages and medical responses in the 2011 off the Pacific coast of Tohoku Earthquake (in Japanese)

International Atomic Energy Agency (2002a) Radiation emergency medical preparedness and response, module II. In: Emergency preparedness and response: medical preparedness and response, EPR-MEDICAL-T. IAEA, Vienna

International Atomic Energy Agency (2002b) Acute radiation syndrome: clinical picture, diagnosis and treatment, module XI. In: Emergency preparedness and response: medical preparedness and response, EPR-MEDICAL-T. IAEA, Vienna

International Atomic Energy Agency (2002c) Emergency medical management on site and at pre-hospital level, module XVI. In: Emergency preparedness and response: medical preparedness and response, EPR-MEDICAL-T. IAEA, Vienna

International Atomic Energy Agency (2002d) Planning the medical response to radiological accidents, module XXII. In: Emergency preparedness and response: medical preparedness and response, EPR-MEDICAL-T. IAEA, Vienna

International Atomic Energy Agency (2005) Emergency preparedness and response: generic procedures for medical response during a nuclear or radiological emergency, EPR-MEDICAL. IAEA, Vienna

International Atomic Energy Agency (2006) Emergency preparedness and response: manual for first responders to a radiological emergency, EPR-FIRST RESPONDERS. IAEA, Vienna

International Atomic Energy Agency (2011) Radiation protection and safety of radiation sources: international basic safety standards – interim edition general safety requirements part 3. IAEA, Vienna

International Commission on Radiological Protection (2007) The 2007 Recommendations of the International Commission on Radiological Protection, ICRP Publication 103. Ann ICRP 37(2–4):103–122

Ishii M (2011) Japan Medical Association Teams' (JMATs) first operation: responding to the Great Eastern Japan Earthquake. World Med J 57:131–140

JAAM (2013) For the victims of the Great East Japan Earthquake, a letter of thanks presented by the Minister of Health, Labour and Welfare. http://www.jaam.jp/html/info/2013/info-20130329.htm. Accessed 19 July 2013 (in Japanese)

Jackson WL Jr, Gallagher C, Myhand RC, Waselenko JK (2005) Medical management of patients with multiple organ dysfunction arising from acute radiation syndrome. BJR Suppl 27:161–168

Kinugasa K (2012) Health monitoring of disaster prevention workers on-site at the early stage of accident. MOOK IRYOKAGAKU 5:53–57 (in Japanese)

Kondo H, Koido Y, Morino K, Homma M, Otomo Y, Yamamoto Y, Henmi H (2009) Establishing disaster medical assistance teams in Japan. Prehosp Disaster Med 24(6):556–564

Kondo H, Shimada J, Morino K, Tase C, Tominaga T, Tatsuzaki H, Akashi M, Tanigawa K, Iwasaki Y, Ichihara M, Kohayagawa Y, Koido Y (2011) Activities of the disaster medical assistance team (DMAT) in response to the TEPCO Fukushima nuclear power plant accident. J Nat Inst Public Health 60:502–509 (in Japanese)

Lataillade JJ, Doucet C, Bey E et al (2007) New approach to radiation burn treatment by dosimetry-guided surgery combined with autologous mesenchymal stem cell therapy. Regen Med 2(5):785–794

Math SB, John JP, Girimaji SC, Benegal V, Sunny B, Krishnakanth K, Kumar U, Hamza A, Tandon S, Jangam K, Meena KS, Chandramukhi B, Nagaraja D (2008) Comparative study of psychiatric morbidity among the displaced and non-displaced populations in the Andaman and Nicobar Islands following the tsunami. Prehosp Disaster Med 23(1):29–34

Morimura N, Asari Y, Yamaguchi Y, Asanuma K, Tase C, Sakamoto T, Aruga T; Members of the Japanese Association for Acute Medicine, Emergency, Task Force on the Fukushima Nuclear Power Plant Accident (JAAM-TF-FNPPA) (2012) Emergency/disaster medical support in the restoration project for the Fukushima nuclear power plant accident. Emerg Med J 0:1–6.doi:10.1136/emermed-2012-201629

National Center for Injury Prevention and Control (2010) Interim planning guidance for preparedness and response to a mass casualty event resulting from terrorist use of explosives. Centers for Disease Control and Prevention, Atlanta. http://www.bt.cdc.gov/masscasualties/pdf/cdc_guidance-508.pdf. Accessed 20 July 2013

Nolan JP, Soar J, Zideman DA, Biarent D, Bossaert LL, Deakin C, Koster RW, Wyllie J, Böttiger B, ERC Guidelines Writing Group (2010) European Resuscitation Council Guidelines for Resuscitation 2010 Section 1. Executive summary. Resuscitation 81(10):1219–1276. doi:10.1016/j.resuscitation.2010.08.021

Sun XC, Zhou XF, Chen S, Liu YX, Wang YJ, Zhang W, Gao YC (2013) Clinical characteristics of hypertension among victims in temporary shield district after Wenchuan earthquake in China. Eur Rev Med Pharmacol Sci 17(7):912–916

Tanigawa K, Ohjino M (2013) Testimony of Doctors; initial medical responses in the Fukushima Daiichi nuclear power plant accident. Herusu Shuppan, Tokyo (in Japanese)

Tanigawa K, Hosoi Y, Terasawa S, Kondo H, Asari Y, Shishido F, Tase C, Tominaga T, Tatuzaki H, Iwasaki Y, Hirohashi N, Akashi A, Kamiya K (2011) Lessons learned from the Fukushima Daiichi nuclear power plant accident; the initial 5 days medical activities after the accident. JJAAM 22(9):782–791. doi:10.3893/jjaam.22.782 (in Japanese)

Tanigawa K, Hosoi Y, Hirohashi N, Iwasaki Y, Kamiya K (2012) Loss of life after evacuation: lessons learned from the Fukushima accident. Lancet 379(9819):889–891. doi:10.1016/S0140-6736(12)60384-5

TEPCO (2011) Mid-and-long-term roadmap towards the decommissioning of Fukushima Daiichi nuclear power units 1–4 (in Japanese)

TEPCO (2012) Current status of irradiation dose of the facility workers at Fukushima Daiichi Nuclear Power Station (in Japanese)

The National Diet of Japan (2012) The official report of the Fukushima Nuclear Accident Independent Investigation Commission: executive summary. The National Diet of Japan, Japan

The Reconstruction Agency of Japan (2012) Report on disaster related death in the Great East Japan earthquake. http://www.reconstruction.go.jp/topics/20120821_shinsaikanrenshihoukoku.pdf. Accessed 20 July 2013 (in Japanese)

Trauma Training Course Developing Committee of JAST & JAAM (2002) Initial trauma management guideline. JATEC. Herusu shuppan, Tokyo (in Japanese)

Ueda S, Hanzawa K, Shibata M, Suzuki S (2012) High prevalence of deep vein thrombosis in tsunami-flooded shelters established after the great East-Japan earthquake. Tohoku J Exp Med 227(3):199–202 (in Japanese)

Valentin J, International Commission on Radiological Protection (2005) Protecting people against radiation exposure in the event of a radiological attack. A report of The International Commission on Radiological Protection. Ann ICRP 35(1):1–110

Yamamoto S (1993) Considerations in disaster prevention for nuclear power plant accidents: roles of the local government and citizens. Katsura Shobo, Toyama (in Japanese)

Yasumura S, Goto A, Yamazaki S, Reich MR (2013) Excess mortality among relocated institutionalized elderly after the Fukushima nuclear disaster. Public Health 127(2):186–188. doi:10.1016/j.puhe.2012.10.019

Disaster Behavioral Health: Psychological Effects of the Fukushima Nuclear Power Plant Accident

4

Masaharu Maeda and Misari Oe

Contents

4.1 Introduction 80
4.2 Behavioral Effects Resulting from the Past Nuclear Accidents 80
4.3 Psychological Consequences of Fukushima Disaster 82
  4.3.1 Posttraumatic Stress Responses 82
  4.3.2 Chronic Anxiety and Guilt 84
  4.3.3 Ambiguous Losses 84
  4.3.4 Separated Families and Communities 85
  4.3.5 Stigma and Self-Stigma 86
4.4 Summary and Implications 87
References 87

Abstract

We reviewed studies regarding the mental health problems of the people who were directly affected by the past three severe nuclear accidents: the Three Mile Island accident, the Chernobyl accident, and the Tokaimura accident. These events brought us many lessons on complicated and long-term

M. Maeda, M.D., Ph.D. (✉)
Department of Neuropsychiatry,
School of Medicine, Kurume University, Fukuoka, Japan

Department of Disaster Psychiatry,
School of Medicine, Fukushima Medical University, Fukushima, Japan
e-mail: maeda_masaharu@kurume-u.ac.jp

M. Oe, M.D., Ph.D.
Division of Health Services,
Institute of Health and Sports Science, Kurume University, Fukuoka, Japan

Department of Neuropsychiatry,
School of Medicine, Kurume University, Fukuoka, Japan
e-mail: oe_misari@kurume-u.ac.jp

K. Tanigawa, R.K. Chhem (eds.), *Radiation Disaster Medicine*,
DOI 10.1007/978-3-319-02216-1_4, © Springer International Publishing Switzerland 2014

sociopsychological effects of the people who met with a nuclear accident. The Fukushima nuclear power plant accident also caused multidimensional behavioral problems of the residents in Fukushima. The various sociopsychological reactions among the Fukushima people can be summarized within five main issues: posttraumatic stress response, chronic anxiety and guilt, ambiguous loss, separated families and communities, and stigma. We should provide the effective intervention to mitigate mothers' anxieties and guilty feelings, dispel the stigma against the Fukushima people, and prevent exhaustion or burnout of the local staff.

4.1 Introduction

The Great East Japan Earthquake brought serious effects on the vast area of Fukushima prefecture. The coastal area in Fukushima, called "Hama-Dori," was heavily affected by the huge tsunami and 1,817 people were presumed dead. However, needless to say, the most serious and long-term effects on the people in Fukushima were caused by the several explosions of the Fukushima Daiichi nuclear power plant after the total electric power loss. The explosions of the three reactor buildings resulted in radioactive contamination in a vast area of the Fukushima prefecture. As the radioactive substances with a long half-life like cesium-134 (^{134}Cs) and cesium-137 (^{137}Cs) widely fell, decontamination efforts using various methods and tools have been tried in many places in Fukushima. Although the Japanese government declared a "cold shutdown" of the plant 9 months after the accident, the process to completely decommission the reactors is estimated to take more than 30 years at least. Even now, there are 17,000 people that were evacuated to temporary houses, 34,000 in municipally subsidized rental houses, and 57,000 living out of Fukushima prefecture.

The nuclear fallouts are both directly and indirectly influencing not only the medical and welfare service but also the politics and the economy of Fukushima. Considering the widespread effects caused by the accident, the psychological problems of the people living in or evacuated from Fukushima should be noted. In this chapter, we will first briefly review past studies regarding the psychological consequences of people experiencing severe nuclear accidents. Subsequently, we will identify the behavioral health problems among the Fukushima people including sociopsychological issues such as public stigma.

4.2 Behavioral Effects Resulting from the Past Nuclear Accidents

Nuclear disasters are very rare events; however, their effects threaten those affected on two levels: from the molecular level to the social level (Christodouleas et al. 2011; Norris et al. 2002a, b). To understand the various psychological impacts affecting the people who have experienced severe nuclear accidents similar to the

Fukushima disaster, we have reviewed past studies related to three nuclear disasters: two very famous nuclear disasters in human history and the first fatal nuclear accident in Japan.

The accident at Three Mile Island (TMI) occurred in 1979 (President's Commission on the accident at Three Mile Island 1979) and was registered as a level 5 on the International Nuclear Event Scale by the International Atomic Energy Agency (IAEA). A series of longitudinal epidemiologic studies was designed to focus on the mental health of the mothers of young children living within ten miles of the plant (Bromet et al. 1982; Fienberg et al. 1985). The concerns about the potential effects of radiation exposure on their children and the mothers' vulnerability to depression were defining reasons as to why they specifically chose those mothers (Fienberg et al. 1985). The results showed that mothers had a stronger risk of experiencing clinical episodes of anxiety and depression during the year following the accident (Bromet et al. 1982). The results from cluster analysis of the same group 10 years following the accident showed two major subgroups of women: those whose temporal profiles were either (a) stable and at a low, clinically nonsignificant psychiatric symptom level across all measurements points (65 % of the sample) or (b) at consistently elevated levels of distress (35 % of the sample) (Dew and Bromet 1993). Multivariate analyses indicated that the pre-accident characteristics, as well as the parameters reflecting the respondents' initial involvement along with the reactions to the accident, were important for distinguishing between the women within the two temporal profile groups (Dew and Bromet 1993). Meanwhile, another study by Prince-Embury and Rooney (1995) revealed that an increased lack of control, a lack of faith in the radiation experts, and an increased fear of developing cancer were observed among the residents following the restart of the nuclear-powered generator.

Other studies on the psychological impacts of nuclear plant workers were conducted by Kasl et al. (1981a, b), and the results demonstrated that the workers of the TMI reactor reported experiencing recurring periods of anger, extreme anxiety, and other varying psychophysiological symptoms at the time of the accident. Six months after the accident, the rate of demoralization was greater primarily among the TMI non-supervisory workers.

The Chernobyl disaster was the first level 7 disaster on IAEA's scale. Although the radiation reached fatal levels, and some 300,000 residents were relocated, the Chernobyl Forum Report from the twentieth anniversary of the Chernobyl event concluded that the mental health effects were the most significant public health consequence of the accident (The Chernobyl Forum 2006; Bromet and Havenaar 2007; Bromet et al. 2011). The cleanup workers showed an increased suicide rate over a longer period of time (Rahu et al. 2006), and the male liquidators complained more often about depression, anxiety disorders, posttraumatic stress disorder (PTSD), suicide ideation, and severe headaches than the control group (Loganovsky et al 2008).

The results of the studies on the influence of the cognitive functioning of the exposed infants are still inconsistent (Bromet et al. 2011); one study showed that Chernobyl did not influence the cognitive functioning of exposed infants in the long term, though many evacuee mothers believed that their offspring had memory problems (Taormina et al. 2008). General population studies also reported a high prevalence rate of depression and PTSD especially among mothers with young children (Bromet et al. 2011).

In Tokaimura, Japan, the criticality accident occurred in a uranium reprocessing facility operated by JCO, the Japanese nuclear company, on 30 September 1999 (IAEA 1999). This resulted in the deaths of two JCO staff members and the evacuation of 161 residents. This accident, which was ranked a level 4 on the IAEA's scale, was considered the worst civilian nuclear radiation accident in Japan prior to the Fukushima Daiichi nuclear power plant accident of 2011.

Following the Tokaimura accident, Japanese psychiatrists began performing consultations of the 59 residents 2–4 weeks after the disaster and found that they complained about concerns of their physical health, anxiety, insomnia, and irritability (Tomita and Nakajima 1999). Furthermore, they also found that mothers with child were concerned about future risks to their pregnancy and the possible adverse effects on their child, including those who were exposed in utero.

Surveys on the symptoms of posttraumatic stress disorder were also conducted after the interventional seminars for the residents around the site. The topics of the lectures were on PTSD symptoms and related psychological issues, titled "Care of Child (after the accident)." Surveys were also conducted at the consultation center (Konishi and Inamoto 1999), and a screening questionnaire of PTSD symptoms (the impact of events scale-revised (IES-R)) was also performed (Asukai et al. 2002). Among the 424 event participants, 31 residents (7.2 %) were considered part of the high-risk group. Meanwhile, 47.5 % ($n=19$) of the consultation center visitors ($n=40$) were placed in the high-risk group. They also revealed that the close proximity and the subjective threat of death had also influenced the IES-R score.

These studies, which addressed the psychological issues in the nuclear crisis in Japan for the first time, brought important findings which can help us to understand the victim's experience after a severe nuclear accident like the Fukushima disaster.

4.3 Psychological Consequences of Fukushima Disaster

There were very complicated psychological impacts on the Fukushima people after the nuclear crisis. We demonstrate five main features as seen in Table 4.1.

4.3.1 Posttraumatic Stress Responses

When the first explosion of the plant occurred following the earthquakes and tsunami, most people, even those who lived near the plant, did not expect such a serious nuclear crisis to happen. They were so poorly prepared for such a crisis that they fell into a panic. The lack of information from the government about the accident spurred the people further. Amid the confusion, most of the

Table 4.1 Features of psychological impact on the Fukushima people after the accident

Psychological impact	Features
Posttraumatic stress responses	Traumatic memories of plant explosion and evacuation Hyperarousal Reexperiencing symptoms
Chronic anxiety and guilt	Fear of radioactive exposure, especially in the case of parents with young children Negative influence on children's development Guilt about abandoning friends and neighbors
Ambiguous loss experience	Loss of home through evacuation rather than damage Uncertainty of nuclear accident evacuees about returning home
Separated families/ communities	Weakened resilience within community Increased conflicts within and between families Frustration of neighboring cities that take in evacuees
Self-stigma	Discrimination against workers and young women Concealment of history in Fukushima Righteous anger Loss of self-esteem

residents living within 30 km from the plant were trying to escape from their hometown. Although some people initially had been optimistic and refused to leave, most of them were eventually evacuated in fear of the meltdown and radioactive exposure.

Afterwards, the government gradually lifted the residential restriction and some of the evacuees returned to their hometown. However, even until today, they still have traumatic memories about the explosions and their evacuation, which yielded various symptoms of posttraumatic stress disorder (PTSD) such as hyperarousal and reexperiencing symptoms (Maeda 2012). The people returning to their hometown are still worried that another explosion at the plant might occur again in the near future. Their worries and anxieties are likely to make them emotionally unstable and may disturb the return of the evacuees. Even in the coastal areas that contain low air level of cesium (e.g., Minami-Soma City), many evacuees still hesitate to return to their hometown due to their close proximity to the plant. Their hesitation shows that the posttraumatic responses and the worries of another explosion among the evacuees continue to exist.

Three months after the Fukushima accident, Kyutoku et al. (2012) performed an online survey for the people in the Tohoku disaster area and revealed that the level of PTSD symptoms for the earthquake and tsunami was significantly higher than that of the nuclear accident. However, considering that the people living near the plant also lived in the coastal area affected by the disaster, both the tsunami and the nuclear crisis may have given them more fearful experiences than the people solely living far from the plant. In the study of the initial patients visiting psychiatric clinics in Fukushima Prefecture after the disaster, the patients showing PTSD or adjustment disorder were 13.9 % of the total number ($n=1{,}321$) (Miura et al. 2012). Unfortunately, we are not able to precisely estimate the psychiatric influence of the nuclear crisis because of a lack of control group comparisons between the Fukushima

Prefecture patients and other disaster areas. However, it is quite possible that the explosion at the plant gave rise to serious traumatic responses among the people living near the plant.

4.3.2 Chronic Anxiety and Guilt

Many of the residents in Fukushima still have chronic anxieties due to the fear of radioactive contamination. Similar to the Three Mile Island in 1979 and the Chernobyl accident in 1986 (Dew and Bromet 1993; Bromet et al. 2011), it is likely that the anxieties among mothers with young children are the highest. The parents are especially nervous about their children possibly touching or handling something dangerous. However, their concerns and the restrictions on their children's outdoor activities could actually have a negative influence on their children's psychological state, as well as their physical development (Save the Children 2012). In a survey of 97 parents visiting a pediatric clinic in Fukushima City 5 months after the disaster, 77.2 % answered that their children became more stressed due to the restrictions on their outdoor activities. 85.1 % also answered that they, if possible, hoped to move to a less affected area (Kitajo 2011).

In addition, many of the parents who stayed behind in Fukushima have experienced guilt for their children and have expressed their fear of being accused of allowing their children to continue to be exposed to radiation by staying in Fukushima (Save the Children 2012). Conversely, the parents who managed to relocate to other areas also had guilt due to the fact that they felt that by escaping their hometown, they abandoned their friends and their neighbors.

It is important to note that the anxieties and guilt from the parents, especially the mothers, are likely to lead to their children's instability. The survey of the pediatric clinic described above (Kitajo 2011) also showed that compared with those before the disaster, the children in Fukushima city tended to be more irritable, more easily offended, more apathetic, and more obsessive. While interacting with their children, their mothers also tended to become more anxious. Furthermore, the mothers' anxieties might elicit negative reactions in their children again, creating a vicious circle. As Raphael (1986) described in her book, these strong interactions between parents and their children are quite common in disasters. Unfortunately, many of the parents and their children in Fukushima are facing these negative intra-familial interactions, such as distress towards other family members.

4.3.3 Ambiguous Losses

In Fukushima, there are still vast areas where people are in danger of radioactive contamination as well as danger from the effects of the tsunami. Over 100,000 people have been evacuated, and many have lost their homes, their jobs, family members, or their sense of community. The elderly people are especially likely to have many difficulties in their readjustment due to the difficulty in changing their jobs and adapting themselves to new circumstances.

Given these losses, we should note that their losses brought by the nuclear crisis are very differently ambiguous from those of the tsunami. Though many houses where the evacuees lived before the disaster are not damaged in appearance, many evacuees are still not allowed to stay or live there by the government's order. Even after the government lifted the restrictions, many evacuees are still hesitant about returning to their homes for several reasons, such as the fear of insufficient decontamination, the difficulty in finding employment, or simply due to uncertainty. On the other hand, the tsunami survivors, despite their great and apparent loss, seemed to have overcome their traumatic experiences faster than the people affected by the accident.

The Fukushima evacuees continue to face a dilemma; they can continue waiting for their hometown to someday become habitable again, but it is unknown when such a situation will occur. Also, this uncertainty has led to difficulties in both compensations and the welfare service. Similar to having a missing loved one (Boss 1999), such ambiguous loss delays the recovery process of the evacuees and may lead to continuing psychiatric problems for the people of Fukushima. In particular, we should pay attention to occurrence of depression or suicide. For example, in Fukushima Prefecture, 32.4 % of the new outpatients having depression or PTSD answered that their symptoms are related to the nuclear accident (Miura et al. 2012). In regard to suicide, several suicidal cases closely related to the nuclear crisis were reported by media, but we have not been able to accurately report on all of these situations.

4.3.4 Separated Families and Communities

In Fukushima, many people were relocated from the affected area both voluntarily and involuntarily. Multiple factors, such as the fear of radioactive exposure, along with residential restrictions, compensations, employment, and/or other personal reasons, divided the residents into two groups: those who decided to relocate and those who did not. Unfortunately, the dissonance between these two groups often arose, which broke the bonds between the original residents.

Generally, if a natural disaster strikes, the bonds and cohesiveness among residents tend to become stronger and, moreover, may enhance the resilience of communities and reduce mental health problems. The past epidemiological study (Kessler et al. 1999) also revealed that the prevalence of PTSD among the people who experienced natural disasters was considerably lower than that among those who experienced other manmade incidents (e.g., motor vehicle accidents, physical assaults, rapes). Japan is known for being affected by a large number of natural disasters, such as earthquakes, tsunamis, or typhoons, and the communities in Japan have developed a sense of resilience from such incidents. However, since the Fukushima accident was essentially a manmade disaster rather than a natural one, the resilience of the communities and the families has weakened.

In Fukushima, there have been three types of discordance which have led to dissonance within both families and the community:

- Family members having different opinions on the physical risk induced by radioactive exposure
- Interfamilial conflicts caused by differences in residential restrictions or compensations
- Frustrations between evacuees and neighboring members taking in large numbers of evacuees (e.g., Iwaki City)

As time passed since the disaster, the souring relationship between the community members and the evacuees worsened due to several reasons: the delinquency of taxes, the unclear period of the evacuees' stay, an increase in population, and the rise in land cost. These three types of discordance have created tension within the population of Fukushima.

4.3.5 Stigma and Self-Stigma

Although the authorities such as the World Health Organization (2013) recommended that the people in Fukushima should not be fearful of the radiation risks in regard to their physical condition, many people are still skeptical. Taking into account the psychosocial burden of the evacuees, it is problematic that there is a public stigma forming through ignorance about the radiation. For example, Shigemura et al. (2012) showed that discrimination was associated with both general psychological distress and posttraumatic responses among the workers engaging in the repair of the destroyed plant. Furthermore, many young women in Fukushima are afraid of how people may look down on them due to assumptions regarding the influence of radiation on pregnancy or on genetic inheritance (Glionna 2012). Some also believe that the women exposed to radiation should not be allowed to marry or reproduce. Unfortunately, due to these misconceptions, many evacuees are hiding the fact that they lived in Fukushima after moving to other prefectures (Save the Children 2012).

This phenomenon reminds us of the atomic bomb survivors of Hiroshima and Nagasaki. They also tried to hide their life history and refused to discuss their experiences of the atomic bombing. In particular, young female survivors also showed the same strong tendency of concealing their experience as those of Fukushima and showed worse psychological symptoms than those of male survivors (Yamada and Izumi 2002).

The self-awareness of both of the atomic bomb survivors and the Fukushima people can be regarded as a "self-stigma" induced by the public stigma related to radioactive contamination. According to the idea of Corrigan et al. (2006), who studied the traits of self-stigma among people with mental disorders, the self-stigma would cause either righteous anger or a loss of self-esteem within the stigmatized people. Also, in the case of Fukushima, such self-stigmas are likely to cause emotional distress within the victims. Given the considerable psychological effects from the self-stigma, dispelling public stigma should be highly prioritized in order to prevent the Fukushima people from further stigmatizing themselves.

4.4 Summary and Implications

In this chapter, we reviewed studies regarding the mental health problems of the people of the nuclear accidents and showed the current behavioral health problems in Fukushima. The various sociopsychological reactions among the Fukushima people can be summarized within five main issues: posttraumatic stress response, chronic anxiety and guilt, ambiguous loss, separated families and communities, and stigma.

Given these complicated problems regarding mental health among the Fukushima people, we should consider the following three approaches. First, we should focus on high-risk groups, such as mothers having young children, and provide effective psychological interventions for them. Second, we should provide adequate risk communication and programs involving the media to dispel the stigma towards the Fukushima people. Lastly, we should provide active support for the medical and welfare of the workers in Fukushima to prevent burnout or exhaustion. By taking these steps towards understanding and resolving these difficulties in a long-term perspective, we can provide strong, relevant aid to those affected by the accident and finally help the Fukushima people overcome the effects of the nuclear power plant accident.

References

Asukai N, Kato H, Kawamura N, Kim Y, Yamamoto K, Kishimoto J, Miyake Y, Nishizono-Maher A (2002) Reliability and validity of the Japanese-language version of the impact of event scale-revised (IES-R-J): four studies of different traumatic events. J Nerv Ment Dis 190(3):175–182

Boss P (1999) Ambiguous loss: learning to live with unresolved grief. Harvard University Press, New York

Bromet EJ, Havenaar JM (2007) Psychological and perceived health effects of the Chernobyl disaster: a 20-year review. Health Phys 93(5):516–521

Bromet EJ, Parkinson DK, Schulberg HC, Dunn LO, Gondek PC (1982) Mental health of residents near the Three Mile Island reactor: a comparative study of selected groups. J Prev Psychiatry 1:225–275

Bromet EJ, Havenaar JM, Guey LT (2011) A 25 year retrospective review of the psychological consequences of the Chernobyl accident. Clin Oncol (R Coll Radiol) 23:297–305

Christodouleas JP, Forrest RD, Ainsley CG, Tochner Z, Hahn SM, Glatstein E (2011) Short-term and long-term health risks of nuclear-power-plant accidents. N Engl J Med 364:2334–2341

Corrigan PW, Watson AC, Barr L (2006) The self–stigma of mental illness: implications for self–esteem and self–efficacy. J Soc Clin Psychol 25(8):875–884

Dew MA, Bromet EJ (1993) Predictors of temporal patterns of psychiatric distress during 10 years following the nuclear accident at Three Mile Island. Soc Psychiatry Psychiatr Epidemiol 28:49–55

Fienberg SE, Bromet EJ, Follmann D, Lambert D, May SM (1985) Longitudinal analysis of categorical epidemiological data: a study of Three Mile Island. Environ Health Perspect 63:241–248

Glionna JM (2012) A year after tsunami, a cloud of distrust hangs over Japan: the Fukushima nuclear disaster has left residents doubting their government, their source of energy, even the food they eat. Los Angeles Times, 11 March. http://articles.latimes.com/2012/mar/11/world/la-fg-japan-quake-trust-20120311. Accessed 20 June 2013

International Atomic Energy Agency (1999) Report on the preliminary fact finding mission following the accident at the nuclear fuel processing facility in Tokaimura, Japan. IAEA, Vienna

Kasl SV, Chisholm RF, Eskenazi B (1981a) The impact of the accident at the Three Mile Island on the behavior and well-being of nuclear workers; part I: perceptions and evaluations, behavioral responses, and work-related attitudes and feelings. Am J Public Health 71(5):472–483

Kasl SV, Chisholm RF, Eskenazi B (1981b) The impact of the accident at the Three Mile Island on the behavior and well-being of nuclear workers; part II: job tension, psychophysiological symptoms, and indices of distress. Am J Public Health 71:484–495

Kessler RC, Borges B, Walters EE et al (1999) Prevalence and risk factors of lifetime suicide attempts in the National Comorbidity Survey. Arch Gen Psychiatry 56:617–626

Kitajo T (2011) Effects of Fukushima nuclear accident on children in Fukushima. Nishoikaiho 42:119–121

Konishi T, Inamoto E (1999) The impacts of the residents near Tokaimura on the mental health consultations after the nuclear accident. In: Yoshikawa T (ed) Health and labour sciences research grant report: PTSD research of residents after the disasters. pp 10–18. http://mhlw-grants.niph.go.jp/niph/search/NIDD00.do?resrchNum=199900066A

Kyutoku Y, Tada R, Umeyama T, Harada K, Kikuchi S, Watanabe E, Liegey-Dougall A, Dan I (2012) Cognitive and psychological reactions of the general population three months after the 2011 Tohoku earthquake and tsunami. Plos One 7(2):e31014

Loganovsky K, Havenaar JM, Tintle NL, Guey LT, Kotov R, Bromet EJ (2008) The mental health of clean-up workers 18 years after the Chernobyl accident. Psychol Med 38:481–488

Maeda M (2012) Difficulties of the staff working at Hibarigaoka Psychiatric Hospital in Minami-Soma. Rinsho-seishinigaku 41:1183–1191

Miura I, Wada A, Itagaki S, Yabe H, Niwa S (2012) Relationship between psychological distress and anxiety/depression following great east Japan earthquake in Fukushima Prefecture. Rinsho-seishinigaku 41:1137–1142

Norris FH, Friedman MJ, Watson PJ, Byrne CM, Diaz E, Kaniasty K (2002a) 60,000 disaster victims speak: part I. An empirical review of the empirical literature, 1981–2001. Psychiatry 65(3):207–239

Norris FH, Friedman MJ, Watson PJ (2002b) 60,000 disaster victims speak: part II. Summary and implications of the disaster mental health research. Psychiatry 65(3):240–260

President's Commission on the accident at Three Mile Island (1979) The need for change, the legacy of TMI: report of the President's Commission on the accident at Three Mile Island. US Government Printing Office, Washington, DC

Prince-Embury S, Rooney JF (1995) Psychological adaptation among residents following restart of Three Mile Island. J Trauma Stress 8(1):47–59

Rahu K, Rahu M, Tekkel M, Bromet E (2006) Suicide risk among Chernobyl cleanup workers in Estonia still increased: an updated cohort study. Ann Epidemiol 16(12):917–919

Raphael B (1986) When disaster strikes: how individuals and communities cope with catastrophe. Basic Books, New York

Save the Children (2012) Fukushima families: children and families affected by Fukushima's nuclear crisis share their concerns one year on. http://www.savethechildren.org/atf/cf/%7B9def2ebe-10ae-432c-9bd0-df91d2eba74a%7D/JAPAN_FUKUSHIMA_FAMILIES_REPORT.PDF. Accessed 25 June 2013

Shigemura J, Tanigawa T, Saito I, Nomura S (2012) Psychological distress in workers at the Fukushima Nuclear Power Plants. JAMA 308(7):667–669

Taormina DP, Rozenblatt S, Guey LT, Gluzman SF, Carlson GA, Havenaar JM, Zakhozha V, Kotov R, Bromet EJ (2008) The Chernobyl accident and cognitive functioning: a follow-up study of infant evacuees at age 19 years. Psychol Med 38(4):489–497

The Chernobyl Forum (2006) Chernobyl's Legacy: health, environmental and socio-economic impacts and recommendations to the Governments of Belarus, the Russian Federation and Ukraine, 2003–2005. pp. 10–11, IAEA, Vienna. http://www.iaea.org/Publications/Booklets/Chernobyl/chernobyl.pdf. Accessed 1 July 2013

Tomita N, Nakajima S (1999) Mental health of the affected residents. In: Yoshikawa T (ed) Health and labour sciences research grant report: PTSD research of residents after the disasters. http://mhlw-grants.niph.go.jp/niph/search/NIDD00.do?resrchNum=199900066A

World Health Organization Report (2013) Health risk assessment from the nuclear accident after the 2011 Great East Japan Earthquake and Tsunami based on a preliminary dose estimation. World Health Organization Report, Geneva. http://www.who.int/ionizing_radiation/chernobyl/WHO%20Report%20on%20Chernobyl%20Health%20Effects%20July%2006.pdf

Yamada M, Izumi S (2002) Psychiatric sequelae in atomic bomb survivors in Hiroshima and Nagasaki two decades after the explosions. Soc Psychiatry Psychiatr Epidemiol 37(9):409–415

Management Perspective: Structure of Radiation Emergency Response in Japan

5

Takako Tominaga, Misao Hachiya, and Makoto Akashi

Contents

5.1 Introduction 90
5.2 History of Radiation Emergency Medicine in Japan 90
5.3 Laws and Regulations Related to Nuclear Disaster Measures 92
5.4 Response System for Radiation Emergency Medicine in Japan 93
5.5 Education, Training, and Exercise/Drills 95
5.6 Temporary House-Visit Program 96
5.7 Public Concerns 96
Conclusion 97
References 97

Abstract

Due to previous local and international radiation incidents, emergency planning and preparedness measures have evolved in Japan. This chapter looks at the history of radiation emergency medicine in Japan and the laws and regulations that are related to radiation disaster countermeasures that have shaped the structure of radiation emergency response in Japan. The response system for radiation emergency medicine gives an overview of prefectural, regional, and national responsibilities of key hospitals that have been designated for radiation emergencies. Additionally, education, training, and drills have been utilized for capacity building in radiation emergency medicine. Radiation emergency

T. Tominaga, M.D., Ph.D. (✉) • M. Hachiya, Ph.D.
Department of Radiation Emergency Medical Assistance Team (REMAT),
National Institute of Radiological Sciences (NIRS), 4-9-1 Anagawa, Inage-ku,
Chiba 263-8555, Japan
e-mail: tominaga@nirs.go.jp

M. Akashi, M.D., Ph.D.
National Institute of Radiological Sciences (NIRS), 4-9-1 Anagawa, Inage-ku,
Chiba 263-8555, Japan
e-mail: akashi@nirs.go.jp

K. Tanigawa, R.K. Chhem (eds.), *Radiation Disaster Medicine*,
DOI 10.1007/978-3-319-02216-1_5, © Springer International Publishing Switzerland 2014

response in Japan in the past has focused on accidents with a small number of workers being heavily exposed in nuclear facilities. However, radiation emergency response for which an entire prefecture or region is involved, as well as radiation knowledge of health professionals, needs to be more developed.

5.1 Introduction

A radiation accident is defined as an unintentional exposure to ionizing radiation or contamination with radionuclides, resulting in possible deleterious effects for the exposed and/or contaminated individuals. Since the discovery of X-rays in 1885 by Roentgen and of radioactivity by Becquerel in 1886, radiation accidents have occurred in society. As early as 1887, Becquerel observed an erythema on his abdomen and ascribed it to radioactive materials. Disaster medicine is performed under circumstances resulting from both natural and man-made disasters. Since multiple members of the general population may be involved in a disaster, management of the public health response to disasters, especially including the health of a total community, is a key issue. Thus, radiation disaster medicine is part of "general" disaster medicine and can be defined as a branch of medicine involved in the management of radiation accidents in which many people might be involved.

Ionizing radiation cannot be seen by the human eye, smelled, heard, or otherwise detected by our normal senses nor do symptoms/signs appear soon after radiation exposure. Moreover, these symptoms/signs are not specific to radiation exposure, and radiation accidents requiring treatment rarely occur. Since opportunities to learn about radiation and its effects are limited, radiation exposure is a highly emotional subject and causes widespread public concern, meaning that the psychological aspects of radiation accidents also require attention.

Medical response to a radiation emergency includes taking appropriate actions to protect yourself and others from radiation. In order to respond to radiation accidents, on the other hand, knowledge of radiation and lessons learned from past accidents must be applied to the fullest. In this section, the structure of the radiation emergency response system in Japan will be discussed, focusing on lessons learned from the accident at Fukushima Daiichi Nuclear Power Plant (NPP) in 2011.

5.2 History of Radiation Emergency Medicine in Japan

During the nuclear test on Bikini Atoll on 1 March 1954, 23 crew members (18–39 years old at the time) of the Lucky Dragon (Daigo Fukuryu Maru) out of Yaizu City, Shizuoka Prefecture, were exposed to radiation. Since that incident, several radiation accidents and nuclear disasters requiring medical care have occurred in Japan: exposure to iridium-192 (^{192}Ir) in 1972, the criticality accident at the nuclear fuel conversion company in Tokaimura in 1999, accidental exposure to X-ray in 2000, and the accident at Fukushima Daiichi Nuclear Power Plant (NPP) of Tokyo Electric Power Co. (TEPCO) in 2011 (Table 5.1) (International Atomic Energy Agency 2012). Until the end of the 1970s, however, no preparation had been made for radiation emergencies in Japan.

Table 5.1 Radiation accidents and incidents in Japan

Year and site	Type of accident	Radiation source	Contents of the accident
1971 Ichibara	Exposure	Ir-192 (industrial use)	A radiation source for nondestructive inspection was lost; a worker picked it up and brought back to his home. A total of six people who visited the home were exposed
1998 Nagasaki	Exposure	Co-60 (industrial use)	Error in retracting source; a worker directly handled the source for 30–60 s
1998 Okinawa	Exposure	Ir-192 (medical use)	Carelessness in touching the source while changing it
1999 Ibaraki	Criticality accident	Uranium (industrial use)	Exceeding limit value of Uranium solution was poured, and then criticality occurred. Three workers were exposed to γ-rays and neutrons and two of them died
1999–2000 Tokyo	Exposure	LINAC (medical use)	Error in inputting dose to computer which controlled therapeutic dose. 23 patients were exposed with exceeding dose
2000 Chiba	Industrial use Exposure	X-ray machine	Three workers intentionally unlocked safety device and their hands were exposed
2000 Gifu, Ibaraki, Mie, Nagano, Saitama	Witness source	Th-232	Monazite ore containing radioactive tritium had been sprayed on the site and repeated failure to report was discovered
2000 Osaka	Contamination	I-125 (laboratory use)	I-125 has been spread at JR Takatsuki Station
2000 Chiba	Inhalation	Natural uranium	Eight workers inhaled natural uranium in the glass company
2001 Tokyo	Exposure	LINAC (medical use)	A man was working on the ceiling and was accidentally exposed to radiation in generation testing
2001 Iwate	Exposure	X-ray machine (educational institutions)	A teacher used the X-ray equipment to show the bones of fingers to students during a class in a high school and then erythema developed in the hand later
2004 Hokkaido	Contamination	F-18 (medical use)	Dealing with medical radionuclide F-18/H_2O, workers were contaminated when they were transferring the nuclide to a plastic bag
2005 Tochigi	Exposure	X-ray machine (industrial use)	In the clean room of an optical equipment company, a worker was accidentally exposed to X-ray from the irradiation device for electrostatic removal of the lens
2008 Ichihara	Case of theft	Ir-192 (industrial use)	A source of nondestructive inspection was stolen and found in the river about 1 month later
2011 Fukushima	Nuclear disaster	I-131, Cs-137, Cs-134, etc.	TEPCO Fukushima Daiichi NPP accident. Large amounts of radionuclides were released to environment and workers, first responders and residents were contaminated and exposed

Accidents/incidents presented in the table are those involving NIRS terms of providing advice, dose assessment, or treatment

After the nuclear accident at Three Mile Island of the USA in 1979, the Central Disaster Prevention Council (CDPC) in the Prime Minister's office reinforced emergency preparedness for dealing with a nuclear power station emergency and issued the report "Urgent Disaster Countermeasures to be taken for Nuclear Facilities by Governmental Agencies" in July 1979. In June 1980, the Nuclear Safety Commission (NSC) of the Japanese government came up with a guideline entitled "Off-site Emergency Planning and Preparedness for Nuclear Power Plants." According to this guideline, the National Institute of Radiological Sciences (NIRS) was selected as a radiation emergency hospital for receiving victims heavily exposed to radiation and/or contaminated with radionuclides due to nuclear or radiological accidents. Not only radiation accidents at Chernobyl, Ukraine, in 1986 and Goiania, Brazil, in 1987 but also the Great Hanshin-Awaji Earthquake in 1995 and fire and explosion at Bituminization Demonstration Facility of Power Reactor and Nuclear Fuel Development Corporation (PNC), Ibaraki Prefecture, in 1997 necessitated further strengthening of the preparedness and planning. In 1999, a criticality accident occurred; three workers were overexposed to γ-rays and neutrons and two of them died of failure of multiple organs due to acute radiation syndrome (ARS) (Akashi et al. 2001). In 2000, the Basic Plan for Disaster was revised and NSC published a report entitled "The Role of Radiation Emergency Medicine" in 2001 (NSC 2001). This report was presented with the aim of saving lives, and it focused on the medical system for small numbers of victims who might become heavily exposed in nuclear facilities. Therefore, responding countermeasures to accidents or disasters involving a large number of residents remained unclear. Thus, there was an urgent need of surge capacity for such a large-scale disaster or a combination disaster, such as natural and man-made disaster (Akashi et al. 2010). This combined disaster occurred at the TEPCO Fukushima Daiichi NPP.

5.3 Laws and Regulations Related to Nuclear Disaster Measures

Countermeasures for nuclear disasters in Japan were contained in "The Basic Disaster Prevention Plan" and "The Basic Act on Disaster Control Measures." Considering lessons learned from the criticality accident at the JCO uranium-processing plant in 1999, "The Basic Disaster Prevention Plan" was revised. The revised plan included responses to facilities for processing, storage and disposal, and transportation of nuclear fuel, in addition to the conventional nuclear power plants and reprocessing facilities. Lessons learned from this accident also led to the establishment of the Act on Special Measures Concerning Nuclear Emergency Preparedness in December 1999. However, based on the nuclear accidents at the Fukushima NPPs, in June 2013 we further revised the laws and regulations mentioned above (Nuclear Regulation Authority (NRA) of Japan 2013).

5.4 Response System for Radiation Emergency Medicine in Japan

Before the Fukushima accident, Japan had 54 operational nuclear reactors for electricity generation installed in 13 prefectures. Nuclear facilities other than NPP, including research facilities and reprocessing plants, were located in six prefectures. Aomori, Ibaraki, and Fukui prefectures have both NPPs and other nuclear facilities, while Kyoto, Tottori, and Nagasaki prefectures are adjacent to nuclear facilities in neighboring prefectures. The response system for radiation emergency medicine had already been established in these 19 prefectures prior to the Fukushima accident (Fig. 5.1).

The report of NSC, as mentioned in the previous section, showed that treatment of patients accidentally exposed and/or contaminated should be performed at three levels of radiation emergency hospitals (Fig. 5.2 and Table 5.2).

NIRS has also been designated as the national center of radiation emergency medicine in Japan besides being a tertiary hospital, providing direct or consultative services to local governments and hospitals. Therefore, NIRS was seeking to improve ties with cooperating hospitals and experts on radiation emergency medicine in "The Radiation Emergency Medical Network Council" and to enable cooperation in radiation emergency medicine with external special organizations for

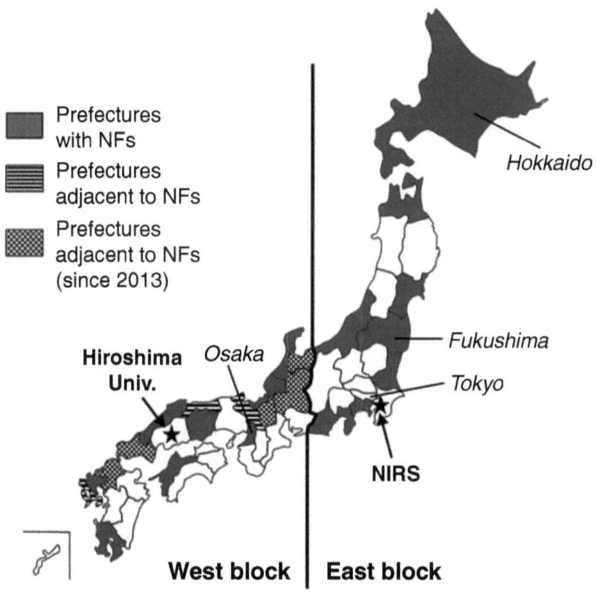

Fig. 5.1 Prefectures with a response system for radiation emergency medicine in Japan. Prefectures that contain nuclear facilities (NFs) or where response systems of radiation emergencies have been established are shown. The response system has been established in prefectures with or adjacent to NFs in Japan

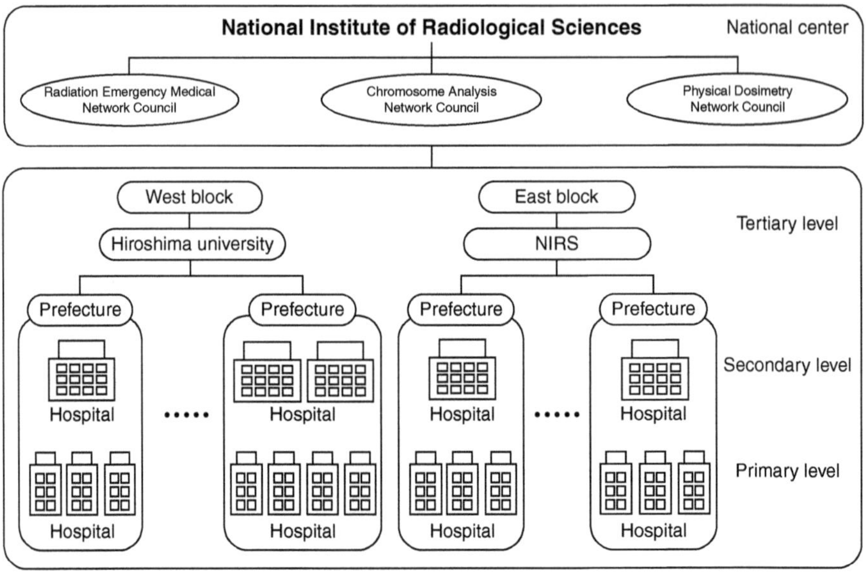

Fig. 5.2 Response system for radiation emergency medicine in Japan. Treatment of patients accidentally exposed and/or contaminated is performed at three levels of radiation emergency hospitals in Japan. Primary- and secondary-level hospitals for radiation emergency medicine are the responsibility of prefectures, while the national government is responsible for the tertiary level of radiation emergency medicine (Nuclear Safety Commission of Japan 2001)

Table 5.2 Three levels of radiation emergency hospitals

Level of radiation emergency hospitals	Description	Function	Designated by
Primary care	Hospital or clinic near nuclear facilities	First aid Primary assessment of contamination with radionuclides Removal of contamination on the body surface	Local government
Secondary care	Local general hospital in local city or town	Medical and radiological triage Decontamination Treatment of local radiation injuries and/or whole body exposure Initiate treatment for internal contamination	Local government
Tertiary care	East block of Japan: NIRS West block of Japan: Hiroshima University Hospital	Specialized medical treatment for acute radiation syndrome, cutaneous radiation syndrome, internal contamination and heavy external contamination Specialized dose assessment for exposure with physical and biological dose assessment	National government

receiving patients requiring specialized medical treatment for radiation exposure. "The Chromosome Analysis Network Council" enabling cytogenetic dose assessments and "The Physical Dosimetry Network Council" enabling physical dose assessments have also been established.

Concerning transportation of victims, exposed and/or contaminated patients are usually transported by ambulance from a nuclear facility to primary- and secondary-level hospitals for radiation emergency medicine in the local area. Helicopters for rescue or disaster can also be used for the transportation of patients, and these measures will be arranged by local governments and fire departments.

When a disaster emergency has been declared by the government, the Japan Self Defense Forces (JSDF) will become involved in long-distance transportation, for example, transportation to NIRS from a secondary hospital.

The revised "The Act on Special Measures Concerning Nuclear Emergency Preparedness" from 2013 shows that the Urgent Protective Action Planning Zone (UPZ) of NPPs, which is the area requiring preparedness for radiation disaster and planning for response, was enlarged from within 10 km from any NPP to 30 km (NRA 2013). Therefore, parts of Gifu, Shiga, Toyama, Yamaguchi, and Fukuoka prefectures, where no nuclear facilities are located, have been designated as UPZs of NPPs.

5.5 Education, Training, and Exercise/Drills

Education, training, and drills are important activities for the capacity building of radiation emergency medicine. Even before the Fukushima accident, a number of training courses were being conducted by radiation-related agencies and organizations for first responders, health care providers, and hospital staff. These training courses provided instructions on basic knowledge and techniques for radiation, radiation protection, handling contaminated patients on-site, at prehospital and hospital, and medical care for exposed and/or contaminated patients. In Japan, central and/or local governments perform annual exercises or drills for radiation emergency or nuclear disaster involving nuclear facilities, police and fire departments, hospitals, and other related organizations/agencies. Then, however, the accident at Fukushima Daiichi NPP revealed that there were a number of problems in terms of medical response to nuclear disaster.

Even prior to the Fukushima accident in 2011, the establishment of a well-organized response system for radiation emergency medicine had been believed to be essential in Japan. However, this accident then revealed inherent problems that included the lack of human resources in radiation emergency medicine rather than an insufficient response system. The smooth transportation of contaminated patients to hospitals and also their receival are vital elements. However, a lack of knowledge about radiation emergency medicine in the personnel who were called upon then resulted in problems including transportation and acceptance of contaminated patients. Such problems may have been based, at least in part, on the fact that opportunities for education in radiation emergency were restricted to personnel in the local governments with or neighboring nuclear facilities before the accident. Therefore, contaminated patients could not be received at a hospital that had not been designated for radiation emergencies and were therefore not ready for radiation emergencies.

5.6 Temporary House-Visit Program

Evacuees who had been living within a 20-km radius from the NPPs had a strong desire to return home temporarily to retrieve their belongings or check on their homes, farms, and businesses. Therefore, temporary house returns of residents were allowed from 10 May 2011. These temporary visits to their homes were limited to 2–5 h to keep radiation exposure to 1 mSv or lower. Only two persons per household were permitted per visit. Residents under 15 years old and senior citizens were initially not allowed on house-return visits. In addition, they could not bring out food or farm animals except pets. Later, the residents' vehicles were allowed to be retrieved by the affected owners. To manage these temporary house visits, local governmental officials requested that NIRS send an expert medical team including physicians, nurses, and radiation-protection experts to manage radiation surveys and provide medical care at the contaminated areas in cooperation with Hiroshima and Hirosaki universities and the National Disaster Medical Center. Residents were asked to wear protective gear to prevent contamination when they entered within the area. In the summer, some people developed heat stroke or dehydration because of the protective gear. However, this program was important for residents who had been evacuated and especially in psychological terms. A temporary house-visit program has to be taken into consideration as part of the public response to radiation emergency, and countermeasures for the radiation protection of residents have to be upgraded.

5.7 Public Concerns

Communicating effectively with the public about radiation effects is vital for the response to succeed. We have already learned from many past accidents that misunderstandings and misconceptions cause considerable anxiety, leading to psychological consequences. Radiation accidents can cause medical, psychological, environmental, and economic problems. Scientifically correct information about health issues is important for the prevention of psychological consequences, and explanation of radiation risks and any countermeasures in plain language is a critical part of an effective risk-communication process for the general public. A variety of information about radiation and its effects was provided via many communication channels such as TV, radio, newspapers, websites, hotlines, written materials, and public meetings just after the incident. Therefore, the general public did not understand which information was right or wrong, and this led to considerable confusion. This was due to the fact that basic knowledge to allow understanding of the information was insufficient. In this regard, as an example, some patients refused medical X-ray tests for the simple reason that radiation increases the risk of cancer.

Conclusion

It is vital that correct knowledge about radiation exposure be shared with people involved in radiation emergency. Otherwise, the effectiveness of the medical system for radiation emergency during an incident will be handicapped. Psychological and economic problems can be prevented or at least minimized. We have learned from the Fukushima accident that human resources supported by basic knowledge concerning radiation exposure are absolutely essential.

References

Akashi M, Hirama T, Tanosaki S, Kuroiwa N, Nakagawa K, Tsuji H, Kato H, Yamada S, Kamata T, Kinugasa T, Ariga H, Maekawa K, Suzuki G, Tsujii H (2001) Initial symptoms of acute radiation syndrome in the JCO criticality accident in Tokaimura. J Radiat Res 42(Suppl):S157–S166

Akashi M, Kumagaya K, Kondo H, Hirose Y (2010) Concerns of Disaster Medical Assistance Team (DMAT) members about troubles at the nuclear power plant: experience from the Niigata Chuetsu–Oki earthquake, 16 July 2007, in Japan. Health Phys 98(6):804–809. doi:10.1097/HP.0b013e3181ac924a

International Atomic Energy Agency (2012) EPR-lessons learned, lessons learned from the response to radiation emergencies (1945–2010). IAEA, Vienna

Nuclear Regulation Authority of Japan (2013) The act on special measures concerning nuclear emergency preparedness (in Japanese). http://www.nsr.go.jp/committee/kisei/data/0009_02r.pdf Accessed 20 June 2013

Nuclear Safety Commission of Japan (2001) The role of radiation emergency medicine. NSC, Tokyo

Management Perspective: Structure of Radiation Emergency Response in International Organizations

6

Azura Z. Aziz and Pisith Phlong

Contents

6.1 Introduction 100
6.2 Conventions 100
6.2.1 The Convention on Early Notification of a Nuclear Accident 100
6.2.2 The Convention on Assistance in the Case of a Nuclear Accident or Radiological Emergency 101
6.3 International Organizations 101
6.4 Incident and Emergency Centre 101
6.5 International Emergency Preparedness and Response Framework 105
6.5.1 Joint Radiation Emergency Management Plan of the International Organizations (Joint Plan or JPLAN) 105
6.5.2 Operations Manual for Incident and Emergency Communication (IEComm) ... 105
6.5.3 Response and Assistance Network (RANET) 106
6.6 Contact Personnel in the Case of Radiation Disasters 106
References 107

Abstract

As the consequences of radiation disasters frequently cross transnational boundaries, International Organizations should be prepared for a coordinated international response to radiation disasters. All key international organization partners who have the mandate to respond to radiation accidents are listed, with further information on the Incident and Emergency Centre of the International Atomic Energy Agency. This chapter highlights two important legal conventions for the international preparedness and response framework

A.Z. Aziz, B.Sc. (Hons) • P. Phlong, M.A. (Anthropology) (✉)
Division of Human Health, International Atomic Energy Agency,
Wagramerstrasse 5, 200 Vienna A-1400, Austria
e-mail: n.a.z.abdul-aziz@iaea.org; p.phlong@iaea.org

K. Tanigawa, R.K. Chhem (eds.), *Radiation Disaster Medicine*,
DOI 10.1007/978-3-319-02216-1_6, © Springer International Publishing Switzerland 2014

to radiation disasters. This framework includes protocols and operational arrangements that have been developed and updated for an effective response to radiation emergencies. In the case of a radiation disaster, information on contacting the appropriate international organization through official communication channels is described.

6.1 Introduction

The impact of radiation disasters frequently goes beyond national boundaries, making it essential for international organizations (IO) with relevant responsibilities and expertise in the field of radiation to coordinate a Joint Plan for an international response to radiation disasters. This Joint Plan will be elaborated upon in Sect. 6.5.1. The authors have no intention to do a detailed narrative of these IO due to the abundance of technical documents (also known as TecDocs) and websites by these diverse IO, which provide available information on radiation disaster responses. The purpose of this chapter is instead to compile an inventory of IO with the mandate to address nuclear radiation accidents.

The authors would like to disclaim that all content on the websites, including dictionary, thesaurus, literature, geography and other reference data, is for informational purposes only. The information should not be considered complete and up to date and is not intended to be used in place of a visit, consultation or advice of a legal, medical or any other professional. If needed, the relevant institution should be contacted directly.

6.2 Conventions

The International Atomic Energy Agency (IAEA) has two conventions, which are legal instruments that outline the international preparedness and response framework to radiation disasters, emergencies, threats or incidents.

6.2.1 The Convention on Early Notification of a Nuclear Accident

The Convention on Early Notification of a Nuclear Accident (IAEA 1986a) requires that the affected State Party releases information to the IAEA and other directly affected countries on the location, time, level and nature of radiation release quickly after the occurrence of the radiation disaster, if it has resulted or may result in an international radiation release crossing State boundaries that could be radiologically significant for another State. The affected State Party shall also supplement relevant information on the development of the emergency situation at suitable intervals. The full text of the convention can be found at this URL: http://www.iaea.org/Publications/Documents/Conventions/cenna.html

6.2.2 The Convention on Assistance in the Case of a Nuclear Accident or Radiological Emergency

The Convention on Assistance in the Case of a Nuclear Accident or Radiological Emergency (IAEA 1986b) establishes an international network to facilitate cooperation and assistance among State Parties and with the IAEA for providing experts, equipment and other materials. The State Party may call for assistance to minimize the consequences of radiation releases and to guard from harm to life, property and the environment. The IAEA shall transmit this request without delay to other States and IO for international assistance, if so requested, using the Response and Assistance Network (RANET) process, which will be elaborated upon later in Sect. 6.5.3. The IAEA may also perform an initial assessment of the radiation emergency, embarking on a field mission if necessary and offer its offices or assistance if required. The full text of the convention can be found at this URL: http://www.iaea.org/Publications/Documents/Conventions/cacnare.html

6.3 International Organizations

The primary coordinating IO for the Joint Plan for radiation disasters is the IAEA. The IAEA has been the focal point in the international system for early notification, warning and assessment of the consequences of radiation disasters and response to radiation emergency situations in accordance with the relevant conventions. All key international partners who have the mandate to respond to radiation accidents and are cooperating in the Joint Plan are as listed in the Table 6.1, with their websites and contact details for more information.

6.4 Incident and Emergency Centre

The Incident and Emergency Centre (IEC) of the IAEA has been set up as the global focal point for readiness and response to radiation disasters and incidents, irrespective of their cause (IAEA 2013a). IAEA's emergency response capabilities were enhanced after the Chernobyl accident, but IEC itself was established in 2005 as an integrated centre within the IAEA to coordinate globally the exchange of information and knowledge sharing and international assistance in responding to radiation disasters and threats.

The Incident and Emergency System is a contact point that is available 24 h a day, 7 days a week for notification and requests for assistance in radiation incidents. On-call officers include an emergency response manager, a radiation safety specialist, a nuclear security specialist and a public information officer. The IEC has rapid communications arrangements to over 200 contact points that include 173 Member States and intergovernmental organizations and an additional 120 Permanent Missions. More information can be found on the IEC Website: http://www-ns.iaea.org/tech-areas/emergency/incident-emergency-centre.asp

Table 6.1 Key international organizations

International organization	Contact information	Description
International Atomic Energy Agency (IAEA)	Address: Vienna International Centre, P.O. Box 100 A-1400 Vienna, Austria, Tel.: + 431 2600-0, Fax: + 431 2600-7, E-mail: Official.Mail@iaea.org, Website: www.iaea.org	"The IAEA is the world's centre of cooperation in the nuclear field. It was set up as the world's 'Atoms for Peace' organization in 1957 within the United Nations family. The Agency works with its Member States and multiple partners worldwide to promote safe, secure and peaceful nuclear technologies" (IAEA n.d.). The role of IAEA is to promptly inform States Parties, Member States and IO about a nuclear accident or radiological emergency, to facilitate prompt assistance to minimize consequences and to protect life, to facilitate cooperation between State Parties and to transmit a request for assistance to other States and international organizations (IAEA 2010a)
World Health Organization (WHO)	Address: Avenue Appia 20 1211 Geneva 27 Switzerland, Tel.: + 41 22 791 21 11, Fax: + 41 22 791 31 11, Website: www.who.int/	"WHO is the directing and coordinating authority for health within the United Nations system. It is responsible for providing leadership on global health matters, shaping the health research agenda, setting norms and standards, articulating evidence-based policy options, providing technical support to countries and monitoring and assessing health trends" (WHO n.d. a). It works closely with the IAEA with regard to readiness and response to nuclear accidents and radiological emergencies. Its principal role in radiation disasters is to provide medical assistance to victims of such events where severe radiation exposure has occurred and coordinate international public health matters (WHO n.d. b)
Food and Agricultural Organization (FAO)	Address: Viale delle Terme di Caracalla 00153 Rome, Italy, Tel.: + 39 06 57051, Fax: + 39 06 570 53152, E-mail: FAO-HQ@fao.org, Website: www.fao.org	"FAO's mandate is to achieve food security for all and to make sure people have regular access to enough high-quality food to lead active, healthy lives". It also works to "raise levels of nutrition, improve agricultural productivity, better the lives of rural populations and contribute to the growth of the world economy" (FAO n.d.). Its role is to "monitor and evaluate the world food security situation"; to "advise governments on measures to be taken in terms of agricultural, fisheries and forestry practices; to minimize the impact of radionuclides; and to develop emergency procedures for alternative agricultural practices and for decontamination of agricultural, fisheries and forestry products, soil and water". It also works to "provide related assistance upon the request or acceptance of governments, without prejudice to the national competence of each of its Member States" (IAEA 2010a)

Nuclear Energy Agency (NEA)	Address: Le Seine Saint-Germain 12, boulevard des Îles 92130 Issy-les-Moulineaux France, Tel.: + 33 1 45 24 82 00, Fax: + 33 1 45 24 11 10, E-mail: nea@oecd-nea.org, Website: www.oecd-nea.org	"The Nuclear Energy Agency (NEA) is a specialized agency within the Organization for Economic Cooperation and Development (OECD), an intergovernmental organization of industrialized countries. The NEA's mission is to assist its member countries in maintaining and further developing, through international cooperation, the scientific, technological and legal bases required for a safe, environmentally friendly and economical use of nuclear energy for peaceful purposes" (NEA 2013). It works to "assist member countries in the regulation and implementation of the system of radiological protection", improve high safety standards in the utilization of nuclear energy and develop "safe, sustainable and societally acceptable strategies" to manage all kinds of radioactive materials (NEA 2011, 2012). It also provides a forum for emergency response experts to share information and experience in every aspect of emergency management systems (IAEA 2010a)
United Nations Environment Programme (UNEP)	Address: United Nations Avenue, Gigiri P.O. Box 30552, 00100 Nairobi, Kenya, Tel.: 254–20 7621234, Fax: 254–20 7624489/90, E-mail: unepinfo@unep.org, Website: http://www.unep.org/	"UNEP, established in 1972, is the voice for the environment within the United Nations system. UNEP acts as a catalyst, advocate, educator and facilitator to promote the wise use and sustainable development of the global environment" (UNEP n.d.). In collaboration with the UN Office for the Coordination of Humanitarian Affairs (OCHA), it forms the Joint UNEP/OCHA Environment Unit which has a role to quickly mobilize and coordinate emergency assistance and response resources to countries dealing with environmental emergencies and natural disasters with significant environmental impacts, including radiological emergencies (IAEA 2010a)
United Nations Scientific Committee on the Effects of Atomic Radiation (UNSCEAR)	Address: UNSCEAR secretariat United Nations Vienna International Centre P.O. Box 500 A-1400 Vienna, Austria, Tel.: + 43 1 26060 4330, Fax: + 43 1 26060 5902, Website: www.unscear.org	"UNSCEAR was established by the General Assembly of the United Nations in 1955. Its mandate in the United Nations system is to assess global levels and effects of exposure to ionizing radiation and report it to the General Assembly" (UNSCEAR 2013). UNSCEAR receives and assembles radiological information from States Members of the UN or members of the specialized agencies about levels of ionizing radiation and radioactivity in the environment, then reviews important problems in the field of ionizing radiation and reports thereon to the General Assembly (IAEA 2010)
United Nations Office for the Coordination of Humanitarian Affairs (OCHA)	Address: OCHA Emergency Services Branch Palais des Nations, Office D-114 CH-1211 Geneva 10 Switzerland, Tel.: + 41 (22) 917 1234, Fax: + 41 (22) 917 0023, E-mail: ochaunep@un.org, Website: www.unocha.org	"The Office for the Coordination of Humanitarian Affairs (OCHA) is part of the United Nations Secretariat and is headed by the Emergency Relief Coordinator, who has the mandate to coordinate UN assistance in humanitarian crises that go beyond the capacity and mandate of any single UN agency". OCHA has the role to process requests from affected Member States for emergency assistance that need a coordinated response, to "maintain an overview of all emergencies through the systematic pooling and analysis of early warning information" and to "organize, in consultation with the government of the affected country, a joint inter-agency needs assessment mission" (IAEA 2010a)

(continued)

Table 6.1 (continued)

International organization	Contact information	Description
The World Meteorological Organization (WMO)	Address: 7bis, avenue de la Paix, Case postale No. 2300 CH-1211 Geneva 2, Switzerland, Tel.: + 41 (0) 22 7308111, Fax: + 41 (0) 22 7308181, E-mail: wmo@wmo.int, Website: www.wmo.int	"The World Meteorological Organization (WMO) is a specialized agency of the United Nations. Its vision is to provide world leadership in expertise and international cooperation in weather, climate, hydrology and water resources and related environmental issues and thereby contribute to the safety and well-being of people throughout the world and to the economic benefit of all nations" (WMO n.d.). It has the role to "facilitate prompt assistance in the event of a nuclear accident or radiological emergency to minimize its consequences and to protect life from the effects of radioactive releases" (IAEA 2010a)
International Labour Organization (ILO)	Address: 4 route des Morillons CH-1211 Genève 22 Switzerland, Tel.: + 41 (0) 22 799 6111, Fax: + 41 (0) 22 798 8685, E-mail: ilo@ilo.org, Website: www.ilo.org	"The International Labour Organization (ILO) is devoted to promoting social justice and internationally recognized human and labour rights, pursuing its founding mission that labour peace is essential to prosperity. Today, the ILO helps advance the creation of decent work and the economic and working conditions that give working people and business people a stake in lasting peace, prosperity and progress" (ILO n.d. a). Radiation protection is part of the ILO's action on occupational safety and health uses. The ILO collaborates with other IO to establish international safety standards on occupational radiation protection (ILO n.d. b)

Note: Information used in the table above is taken from the organization's website

6.5 International Emergency Preparedness and Response Framework

There are several protocols and operational arrangements that have been put in place between IAEA, Member States and other IO for a timely, managed, controlled, coordinated and effective response to any radiation emergency within the legal framework of the two abovementioned conventions (IAEA 2013b). These are the *Joint Radiation Emergency Management Plan of the International Organizations*, the *Operations Manual for Incident and Emergency Communication* and the *Response and Assistance Network*.

More detailed information on the international response system can be found at this website: http://www-ns.iaea.org/tech-areas/emergency/international-response-system.asp?s=1&l=4

6.5.1 Joint Radiation Emergency Management Plan of the International Organizations (Joint Plan or JPLAN)

The JPLAN outlines the inter-agency framework for readiness for and response to an actual, potential or perceived radiological incident or emergency (IAEA 2010a). There are many IO partners in this JPLAN and the full text about tasks, roles, responsibilities and procedures of these IO partners to response to radiological incident and emergency can be found at this URL: http://www-pub.iaea.org/MTCD/publications/PDF/EPR-JPLAN_2010_web.pdf

The JPLAN does not impose arrangements between the participating IO; instead, it provides a common understanding of how each IO acts during a response and in making readiness arrangements. The JPLAN is also intended neither to interfere with nor to substitute any emergency response arrangements of Member States or IO. However, all Member States are encouraged to consider these arrangements in their own emergency management plans, wherever appropriate.

6.5.2 Operations Manual for Incident and Emergency Communication (IEComm)

IEComm describes the IAEA's "expectations regarding notification and reporting, the exchange of official information and the timely provision of assistance among the IAEA's Secretariat, its Member States, Parties to the two abovementioned Conventions, relevant IO and other States in events with apparent, potential or perceived radiological consequences that necessitate response actions or that raise media interest and the development of preparedness" (IAEA 2012). The manual gives guidance such that they may develop appropriate arrangements to interface with each other and the IAEA Secretariat. IEComm also contains practical information that is pertinent to invoking these arrangements for emergency notification. The full text of the manual can be found at this URL: http://www-pub.iaea.org/MTCD/publications/PDF/EPR_IEComm-2012_Web.pdf

All Member States are encouraged to use the IEComm arrangements in the provision of relevant information regarding radiological incidents or emergencies, so as to minimize the consequences and to facilitate timely delivery of information and assistance.

6.5.3 Response and Assistance Network (RANET)

IAEA has set up a response system in order to answer to Member States' requests for assistance during a radiological incident or emergency. RANET is a network of Member States that are capable and willing to provide, when requested, specialized assistance by personnel who have been appropriately trained, equipped and qualified with the ability to respond quickly and effectively to radiation incidents. Additionally, RANET aims to facilitate and coordinate the harmonization of emergency assistance and response capabilities and pertinent information exchange and feedback of experience (IAEA 2010b).

RANET does not interfere or affect the cooperation arrangements that have been defined in any bilateral and/or multilateral agreements between Member States. The IEC may, when requested, evaluate the radiological situation and deploy a fact finding Assistance Mission to the requesting state to further assess the radiation emergency, among other responsibilities. The tool on how to request and provide assistance between Member States and IAEA is described in RANET, and the full text of RANET can be found at this URL: http://www-pub.iaea.org/MTCD/publications/PDF/Ranet2010_web.pdf

6.6 Contact Personnel in the Case of Radiation Disasters

Under The Convention on Early Notification of a Nuclear Accident (IAEA 1986a), in the event of a nuclear accident, the State Party involved shall "notify, directly or through the IAEA, those States which are or may be physically affected and the IAEA of the nuclear accident" and provide the States, "directly or through the IAEA, and the IAEA with such available information relevant to minimizing the radiological consequences in those States". Upon receipt of notification from the State Party involved, States Parties, Member States, other States which are or may be physically affected and relevant IO are informed through the IAEA and, upon request, provided with further relevant information. The contact information listed in Table 6.2 is as of June 2013.

Table 6.2 Contact personnel for radiation emergencies (IAEA 2012)

International Atomic Energy Agency	Contact information for radiation emergencies
IAEA Incident and Emergency Centre Routine correspondence: Routine tel.: + 43 1 2600 22026 (or 22745 as backup), Routine fax: + 43 1 26007 29309, Routine email: iec3@iaea.org	Communication in the event of a nuclear or radiological incident or emergency need to be through the arrangements described in IEComm Attachment 1 (available upon request by the officially designated competent authorities and contact points under the Early Notification Convention and the Assistance Convention) Contact details, communication arrangements and all official contact points are restricted in their distribution and are available only to designated national warning points, national competent authorities and relevant international organizations. E-mail should not be used as the communication channel for the initial notification or advisory messages, for reporting a change of emergency class or for requesting assistance

Note: Information used in the table above is taken from the organization's website

Acknowledgments The authors would like to thank Ms. Elena Buglova, IEC, IAEA, for her valuable comments and input to this chapter.

References

FAO (n.d.) About FAO. http://www.fao.org/about/en/. Accessed 31 May 2013

IAEA (1986a) Convention on early notification of a nuclear accident. http://www.iaea.org/Publications/Documents/Conventions/cenna.html. Accessed 17 June 2013

IAEA (1986b) Convention on assistance in case of a nuclear accident or radiological emergency. http://www.iaea.org/Publications/Documents/Conventions/cacnare.html. Accessed 17 June 2013

IAEA (2010a) Emergency preparedness and response: joint radiation emergency management plan of the International Organizations. IAEA, Vienna

IAEA (2010b) Emergency preparedness and response: IAEA Response and Assistance Net-work. IAEA, Vienna

IAEA (2012) Emergency preparedness and response: operations manual for incident and emergency communication. IAEA, Vienna

IAEA (2013a) Incident and Emergency Centre. http://www-ns.iaea.org/tech-areas/emergency/incident-emergency-centre.asp. Accessed 4 June 2013

IAEA (2013b) International response system. http://www-ns.iaea.org/tech-areas/emergency/international-response-system.asp?s=1&l=4. Accessed 4 June 2013

IAEA (n.d.) About the IAEA. http://www.iaea.org/About/about-iaea.html. Accessed 31 May 2013

ILO (n.d. a) About the ILO: mission and objectives. http://www.ilo.org/global/about-the-ilo/mission-and-objectives/lang--en/index.htm. Accessed 3 June 2013

ILO (n.d. b) Radiation protection. http://www.ilo.org/safework/areasofwork/radiation-protection/lang--en/index.htm. Accessed 4 June 2013

NEA (2011) Nuclear safety and regulation. http://www.oecd-nea.org/nsd/. Accessed 31 May 2013

NEA (2012) Radioactive waste management and decommissioning. http://www.oecd-nea.org/rwm/. Accessed 31 May 2013

NEA (2013) The nuclear energy agency. https://www.oecd-nea.org/nea/. Accessed 31 May 2013

UNEP (n.d.) About UNEP. http://www.unep.org/documents.multilingual/de-fault.asp?DocumentID=43&ArticleID=3301&l=en. Accessed 31 May 2013

United Nations Scientific Committee on the Effects of Atomic Radiation (2013) General assembly. http://www.unscear.org/unscear/en/general_assembly.html. Accessed 3 June 2013

WHO (n.d. a) About WHO. http://www.who.int/about/en/. Accessed 3 June 2013

WHO (n.d. b) Ionizing radiation: radiation accidents and emergencies. http://www.who.int/ionizing_radiation/a_e/en/. Accessed 3 June 2013

WMO (n.d.) WMO's desired outcomes, strategies and associated goals. http://www.wmo.int/pages/about/vision_en.html. Accessed 4 June 2013

Radiation Disaster Medicine Curriculum Revisited in a Post-Fukushima Context

7

Rethy Kieth Chhem, Azura Z. Aziz, and Gregory K. Clancey

Contents

7.1 Background 110
7.2 Introduction 111
7.3 Emerging Issues 111
7.4 Strategic Response from NAHU/IAEA 112
7.5 Theoretical Framework: Science and Technology Studies (STS) Approach 113
7.6 Existing Academic Responses to Knowledge Gaps Arising from the Fukushima Accident 114
7.7 Project NA9/16: "Enhancing Radiation Medicine Education by Building Capacity of Health Professionals and Medical Students" 115
7.8 Project NA9/17: "Strengthening Research Cooperation in Radiation Disaster Medicine Including Posttraumatic Stress Disorders" 116
Conclusion 117
References 118

R.K. Chhem, M.D., Ph.D. (Edu), Ph.D. (His) (✉)
Division of Human Health, International Atomic Energy Agency, Wagramerstrasse 5, 200, Vienna A-1400, Austria

Fukushima Medical University, Fukushima, Japan

Hiroshima University, Hiroshima, Japan

Nagasaki University, Nagasaki, Japan

Institute of History, Philosophy and Ethics of Medicine, Ulm University, Ulm, Germany
e-mail: r.chhem@iaea.org

A.Z. Aziz, B.Sc. (Hons)
Division of Human Health, International Atomic Energy Agency, Vienna, Austria
e-mail: n.a.z.abdul-aziz@iaea.org

G.K. Clancey, Ph.D.
Asia Research Institute, National University of Singapore, Singapore, Singapore

Tembusu College, National University of Singapore, Singapore, Singapore
e-mail: hisgkc@nus.edu.sg

K. Tanigawa, R.K. Chhem (eds.), *Radiation Disaster Medicine*,
DOI 10.1007/978-3-319-02216-1_7, © Springer International Publishing Switzerland 2014

Abstract

The International Atomic Energy Agency (IAEA) has a distinctive mandate to "accelerate and enlarge the contribution of atomic energy to peace, health, and prosperity throughout the world." The Division of Human Health (NAHU) of the IAEA recognizes education and research as key components of "readiness, response, and recovery" with respect to a major nuclear accident. In this chapter, we address ongoing efforts of NAHU to foster a more comprehensive Science and Technology Studies (STS) approach to creating and mobilizing new knowledge of radiation medicine. This includes promoting collaborative education and research programs and policies based on lessons from the Fukushima accident. NAHU is playing an instrumental role in this process. We discuss results from a consultancy meeting on "Global Radiation Medicine: Educational Challenges for Academia," which used a focus group methodology. Two STS-oriented projects are being implemented as an outcome of this meeting. The first aims to enhance global radiation medicine education by building capacity among physicians, health professionals, and medical students. The second project aims to strengthen research cooperation in radiation disaster medicine, including the psychosocial consequences of disasters. NAHU mobilizes both international and Japanese STS and disaster studies experts as a way to integrate outsider and insider perspectives on the Fukushima recovery process and draw on the contributions of health professionals, medical students, and specialists from relevant fields such as sociology, anthropology, history, and psychology.

7.1 Background

At 2.46 p.m. Japan Standard Time (JST) on 11 March 2011, the Great East Japan earthquake of magnitude 9.0 triggered powerful tsunamis up to 40 m high. The earthquakes and tsunamis caused several power plant accidents, most significantly at the Fukushima Daiichi nuclear power plant, where 14-m tsunami waves flooded rooms housing emergency generators. These were meant to supply electricity to pumps cooling the reactors. With the pumps stopped, the three reactors overheated, leading to a full nuclear meltdown.

Subsequent hydrogen explosions occurring at the plant released radioactive material into the atmosphere, which amounted to 1.6×10^{17} Becquerels (Bq) of iodone-131 (^{131}I), 1.8×10^{16} Bq of cesium-134 (^{134}Cs), and 1.5×10^{16} Bq of cesium-137 (^{137}Cs) (Nuclear and Industrial Safety Agency 2011). These radiation leaks caused the evacuation of about 200,000 people within 20 km of the plant by 15 March 2011. The accident rating was raised from Level 5 to Level 7 on the International Nuclear Event Scale (INES) on 12 April 2011, which is the highest possible level, as radiation leakage was still ongoing (Wheeler and Dotson 2011).

The earthquake, tsunami, and nuclear accident caused almost 16,000 deaths, although no deaths have been attributed to acute radiation exposure (Hamblin 2012). About half a million people became homeless, including those that had to be evacuated due to their proximity to nuclear power plants. 1.9 million people faced a shortage of electricity and 1.5 million experienced a shortage of water (NPR Staff and Wires 2011). Additionally, differential information from the authorities and experts, which is typical of post-disaster scenarios, resulted in an erosion of public trust (Brumfiel and Fuyuno 2012), the destruction of infrastructure, and damage to the administrative functions of local governments. A lack of nuclear emergency preparedness hampered the immediate humanitarian aid and medical response in the region surrounding the Fukushima Daiichi nuclear power plant (The Economist 2011; Hayashi and Tomita 2012). The Fukushima accident had, in other words, wide-impacting economic, political, social, technological, and psychological consequences. The Japanese, particularly those in Fukushima prefecture, found themselves living in an environment of uncertainty and anxiety about their futures.

7.2 Introduction

The International Atomic Energy Agency (IAEA) has a distinctive mandate to "accelerate and enlarge the contribution of atomic energy to peace, health, prosperity throughout the world," as stated in the Statute of the IAEA, Article II (IAEA 1957). The Division of Human Health (NAHU) of the IAEA recognizes that education and research are key components of "readiness, response, and recovery" in tackling future nuclear accidents. In order to create and mobilize new knowledge of radiation medicine, NAHU is calling for a more comprehensive Science and Technology Studies (STS) approach to be integrated into collaborative education and research programs and policy implementations as based on lessons from the Fukushima accident.

7.3 Emerging Issues

NAHU has observed some emergent issues in the relationship between nuclear accidents and society. First, there is a "crisis in expertise" in the lack of trust in expert advice, particularly in Japan but also globally. This is partly due to conflicting advice (if not perceptions) by experts from different fields, backgrounds, and countries, amidst an evolving call for more transparency about the risks and dangers of radiation from nuclear power plants. The Internet and the ubiquity of social media mean that there is no central source for trusted information and rumors or misinformation can spread widely and quickly, to be archived alongside accurate and useful information. Discussion about radiation and health has also become intermingled with national and international debates about the future of nuclear power, with political positions influencing the construction and delivery of health information (Clancey 2012a). All of this creates a very different context for disseminating public health information about radiation in the aftermath of an accident or disaster.

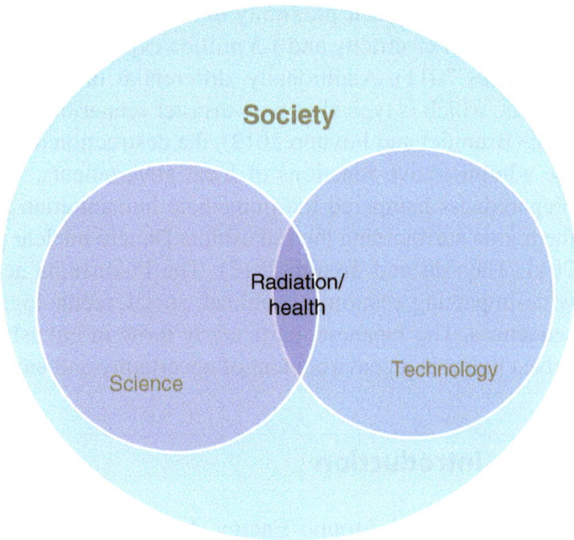

Fig. 7.1 "Radiation-society interaction" conceptual framework

7.4 Strategic Response from NAHU/IAEA

Based on these and other observations, NAHU decided to initiate a strategic response by revisiting radiation disaster medicine education. We did so through the organization of an interdisciplinary consultancy meeting entitled "Global Radiation Medicine: Educational Challenges for Academia," summarized in a report to the IAEA by Clancey (2012a). This is the first time that such an initiative on radiation disaster medicine has ever taken a comprehensive and socially informed approach, with the involvement of international experts from not only radiation medicine but also the social sciences and the humanities.

We invited STS scholars to engage in a project whose outcomes may also have broad implications for STS policies and practices. Throughout this consultancy meeting, NAHU played an instrumental role in calling for a more comprehensive and formalized STS approach to creating and mobilizing new knowledge of radiation medicine. This consultancy meeting was held in Vienna in October 2012 and reviewed the status of educational initiatives in what we called a "radiation-society interaction" context. This discussion principally considered the Fukushima accident recovery efforts and judged their potential contribution to a globally relevant curriculum on radiation disaster medicine. The "radiation-society interaction" context involves the intersection between radiation, health, and society using an STS framework, seen in Fig. 7.1. Radiation and health can be examined from the intersection of science and technology, with all the different elements embedded within society and its values.

As a result of the consultancy meeting, NAHU is implementing two STS-oriented projects over two years starting in 2013. These two projects operate on two fronts: (1) the enhancement of radiation medicine education by building capacity of physicians, health professionals, and medical students and (2) the strengthening of research cooperation in radiation disaster medicine including the psychosocial consequences of disasters. These projects are collaborative between the IAEA and Fukushima Medical University (FMU) (Practical Arrangements 2012) and include conferences, consultancy meetings, symposiums, and research activities.

7.5 Theoretical Framework: Science and Technology Studies (STS) Approach

The Science and Technology Studies (STS) approach examines the inextricable connections and relationships between the different realms of science, technology, and society, as informed by relevant disciplines in the social sciences and humanities such as sociology, history, anthropology, and psychology. Technoscientific disasters can reveal emergent problems and knowledge gaps in social and physical infrastructure and generate intense debate among an expanding number of stakeholders (Clancey 2012b).

The scientific and technical expertise required to manage the aftermath of the Fukushima accident may or may not be sufficient, but expertise in the social and humanistic dimensions of scientific and technical knowledge has certainly been underdeveloped and would clearly add value to the recovery process. By examining the post-Fukushima accident recovery context from an STS perspective, a better understanding of how citizens, medical institutions, governmental institutions, nuclear industry, and radiation experts shape and are shaped by the social, cultural, and political forces of science and can be analyzed (Fortun and Frickel 2012; Clancey 2012b).

"Radiation-society interaction" problems have partly stemmed from diverse advice and statements from experts, official sources, and the media, bringing about widespread distrust in "expert advice" (Brumfiel and Fuyuno 2012; Clancey 2012a). Straight after the hydrogen explosions released radioactive material into the atmosphere, varying official statements and radiation readings drove concerned citizens, most of whom only had superficial knowledge of radiation issues, to turn to the internet and social media. Online there was much discussion, but naturally no consensus (and much misinformation) about the effects of radiation on health. The official media played an equally damaging role by creating misleading information regarding internal exposure (Sakai 2011) leading to even greater confusion, radiation anxiety, and uncertainty.

The residents of Japan have a genuine and legitimate desire to be aware and engaged on the subject of radiological effects on human health and what has happened and is happening in Fukushima. However, as they are reluctant to trust official reports or as reports from experts are transmitted in technical jargon, there is a breakdown in communication between the government, experts, and the larger community. The inclusion of STS and science communication for physicians, health professionals, and medical students in the implementation of this project could contribute to improved understanding and communication between health professionals and the populations they serve.

NAHU emphasizes that education, research, and public engagement are key components of "readiness, response, and recovery" in tackling future nuclear accidents. All relevant groups including the national government, local governments, local and foreign experts, medical institutions, and society itself have a part to play in the "readiness, response, and recovery" in the "radiation-society interaction" context. As physicians and health professionals form the team of first responders to nuclear accidents, strengthening radiation medicine education and research that involves elements of STS is vital to preparation for future nuclear accidents. In Sects. 7.7 and 7.8, we discuss the two STS-oriented projects that are being implemented in order to raise these related issues to global attention and to guide policy.

7.6 Existing Academic Responses to Knowledge Gaps Arising from the Fukushima Accident

A sharing of radiation medicine expertise from Hiroshima University, Nagasaki University, the National Institute of Radiological Sciences (NIRS), and Fukushima Medical University (FMU) is especially important due to their experience in radiation specialization. Together, innovative solutions to fill these knowledge gaps have been proposed by academic institutions in the form of curricular and education programs.

Hiroshima University has recognized that the management of radiation disaster recovery requires "global leaders who have comprehensive knowledge of various disciplines" (Kamiya et al. 2012), highlighting the importance of risk communication and radiation education. With the support of Japan's Ministry of Education, Culture, Sports, Science and Technology, Hiroshima University launched a new Ph.D. program in 2011 in radiation disaster recovery studies, called the "Phoenix Leader Education Program for Renaissance from Radiation Disaster" (Okamoto et al. 2012). Phoenix leaders will be educated to respond to radiation disasters in a comprehensive way, protecting individual human lives, the environment, and society.

Similarly, Nagasaki University has generated extensive data and experience from not only caring for atomic bomb victims in Japan but also collaborating in studies on the Chernobyl nuclear accident site and among affected people in Belarus. The university realized the need for trained personnel for radiation risk control and thus launched a Master's course in radiation nursing in 2011 (Takamura 2012). Nurses from the Master's course participated in the medical relief team in the Fukushima accident recovery efforts. Nagasaki University also dispatched radiation emergency medical assistance teams (REMAT) to FMU Hospital after the Fukushima accident (Matsuda 2012) to support the recovery efforts.

FMU initially had only a small number of medical staff who was capable of responding to the needs of Fukushima residents and of addressing radiation and disaster issues related to psychosocial problems. The university's approach was to establish the Education Center for Disaster Medicine and to conduct the Fukushima Health Management Survey to monitor health conditions of Fukushima residents (Yamashita and Kumagai 2012a). Disaster medical seminars are held at the

Education Center for Disaster Medicine to develop radiation-related knowledge among existing medical staff at Fukushima hospitals in the short term and to build capacity of health professionals well-trained in disaster management in the long run (Yamashita and Kumagai 2012b).

NIRS has highlighted the knowledge gap of insufficient widespread basic knowledge and experience in radiation protection in medical education, without which physicians and health professionals will not be able to respond to a nuclear disaster appropriately. In response to this issue, NIRS revised the Guidelines for Medical Education, which is a reference for medical school curricula, on 31 March 2011, just after the Great East Japan earthquake (Akashi 2012). In April 2012, NIRS released a "Reference Document on Education and Self-Study Related to Radiation Medicine in Medical Education," which calls for the inclusion of radiation exposure and protection in all medical curricula (NIRS 2012).

7.7 Project NA9/16: "Enhancing Radiation Medicine Education by Building Capacity of Health Professionals and Medical Students"

This project aims to enhance global radiation medicine education and training of physicians, health professionals, and medical students in radiation disaster management. It was clear from early medical responses at Fukushima Medical University that the physicians and health professionals were medically and psychologically unprepared to handle a nuclear accident, such that they needed to refer to textbooks for basic radiation decontamination procedures and experienced anxiety and confusion due to a dearth of information on the current situation of the Fukushima Daiichi nuclear plant (Hasegawa et al. 2012). Thus, it is essential to build capacity of physicians, health professionals, and medical students in radiation education to ensure that they are medically and psychologically ready for such an eventuality and that they are able to respond effectively to address the radiation anxiety of patients, fellow emergency responders, and relevant citizens. REMAT was able to guide physicians and health professionals, help assemble radiation emergency triage, and conduct radiation risk communication lectures. This highlighted the need to train health professionals, in order to lead and direct response and recovery measures in difficult circumstances such as those faced at FMU Hospital, not only which had little information on the situation outside its walls but whose water supply was cut off and whose food supplies dwindled over time (Matsuda 2012).

In the post-Fukushima context, far-reaching problems that have resulted from the nuclear accident need to be factored into any preparation for future recovery measures. Physicians, health professionals, and medical students should undergo education and training programs that cover the intertwining of medical and psychosocial consequences associated with radiation accidents. These programs are necessarily interdisciplinary and include the issues of psychosocial effects of disaster and communication in an atmosphere of uncertainty and possible mistrust (Clancey 2013).

In July 2013, a small working group met in a plenary session at the Asia-Pacific Science, Technology and Society Network (APSTSN) conference in Singapore to activate and engage with the regional STS community around the topic of "medical and academic responses to the Fukushima nuclear accident." This project has also been instrumental in organizing the very first STS-oriented international conference in Fukushima itself that will take place in November 2013, entitled "Radiation, Health and Society: Post-Fukushima Implications for Health Professional Training" (Clancey 2013). The purpose of the international conference is to share expertise on radiation medical education and STS in the medical curriculum. The emphasis on STS is to create awareness of the value of social science in a medical curriculum.

The implementation of this project will result in positive changes in global radiation medicine education and the harmonization of both national and international capacity building for physicians, health professionals, and medical students. During the course of this project, guides for developing these programs will be prepared and suggested for implementation, for not only the citizens from the areas of Japan affected by the Fukushima accident but also those in other parts of the world where nuclear accidents may happen in the future. It is imperative for there to be international preparedness for radiation-related accidents and their psychosocial consequences. In addition, further strategies for addressing the issue of radiation anxiety and psychosocial effects of disaster will be prepared and suggested for implementation.

7.8 Project NA9/17: "Strengthening Research Cooperation in Radiation Disaster Medicine Including Posttraumatic Stress Disorders"

This project aims to strengthen research capabilities of physicians, health professionals, and medical students from the standpoint of radiation education. In particular, one of the research projects will focus on the psychosocial consequences in the post-Fukushima accident recovery context and will investigate the phenomenon of intergenerational transmission of traumatic experiences.

The first technical meeting of this project was in May 2013 and included Japanese and international experts in the field of radiation and STS. Through this initiative, radiation medicine experts were introduced to STS, and the boundaries and potential contributions of STS in radiation disaster medicine were collectively defined. STS was emphasized to create awareness of the value of social science in the medical curriculum. The participants agreed that the current medical curriculum was inadequate with respect to radiation disaster education and that the abovementioned academic responses could be supplemented with the inclusion of STS elements in medical curricula. Further developments of this project are being planned, including a handbook on "STS for Health Professionals" that will gather STS experts to collect most updated data relevant to the curriculum's needs, as expressed by FMU.

The radiation leak at the Fukushima Daiichi nuclear power plant and the subsequent evacuation of all residents living within a 20 km radius of the plant has resulted in radiation anxiety and post-disaster psychosocial effects. These are due not only to fears about radiation exposure and its long-term effects on their health but to drastic changes in their social and physical environment (Ozawa et al. 2011). Mental health issues affect many Fukushima residents, but more significant are those affecting young children, adolescents, and the elderly. A project focusing on psychosocial consequences of the Fukushima recovery context is being developed and is planned to take place in 2014.

The standpoint of intergenerational trauma indicates contagion and repeated patterns within an affected generation. Within the context of the traumatic experiences and their impact on different generations, the significance of certain behavioral symptoms that transcend generations can be examined through these repeated patterns (Danieli 1998). At this juncture, the relevant case studies on possible intergenerational transference of trauma in the nuclear disaster context are on Chernobyl, Hiroshima, and Nagasaki. A recent study of the grandchildren of Hiroshima and Nagasaki atomic bomb survivors revealed that they are more vulnerable to posttraumatic stress disorders in the wake of the Fukushima accident than those who had no grandparents who lived in Hiroshima or Nagasaki (Palgi et al. 2012). This study would be a good springboard to generate conceptualizations of intergenerational transmissions of traumatic experiences that take into account the specific cultural, historical, and social context surrounding the Fukushima accident. The dearth of intergenerational trauma studies related to nuclear issues gives way to a myriad of different directions in research.

The implementation of this project will fill crucial gaps in the understanding of the type and means of knowledge that are obtained by physicians, health professionals, and medical students from the standpoint of radiation education and also of research into immediate and long-term psychosocial consequences of nuclear disasters. This research will be distributed globally and used to inform related policies.

Conclusion

The Division of Human Health (NAHU) of the IAEA is dedicated to the coordination, creation, and mobilization of new knowledge related to radiation disaster medicine for the benefit of the Japanese population, as well as the populations of all other countries that have or are planning to have nuclear power plants. We recognize that education and research form key elements of "readiness, response, and recovery" to ensure the safety and minimize the risk of nuclear power plants in the case of future nuclear accidents. As the output and consensus from the consultancy meeting in 2012, the projects that are under way aim to enhance collaborative radiation medicine education, and research programs, involving both international and Japanese STS and disaster studies experts, are a way to integrate both outsider and insider perspectives on the Fukushima accident recovery efforts. A more comprehensive STS approach, informed by perspectives from the fields of sociology, history, anthropology, and psychology, among others, would definitely be of aid to physicians, health professionals, and medical students based on post-Fukushima accident lessons.

This groundbreaking initiative will address the key issues in "radiation-society interaction" through conferences, consultancy meetings, workshops, symposiums, and research activities over the course of 2 years (2013–2014) with the goal of raising these matters to global attention and stimulate further global thinking, research, and action that can be incorporated into related policies.

Acknowledgments The authors thank Mr. Soveacha Ros for his helpful comments and editorial assistance.

References

Akashi M (2012) Education and self-study related to radiation medicine in medical education [Powerpoint slides]. Retrieved from consultancy meeting "Global Radiation Medicine: Educational Challenges for Academia"

Brumfiel G, Fuyuno I (2012) Fukushima's legacy of fear. Nature 483(7388):138–140. doi:10.1038.483138a

Clancey G (2012a) Report to IAEA for consultancy meeting "Global Radiation Medicine: Educational Challenges for Academia". Vienna, Oct 29–Nov 2

Clancey G (2012b) An STS approach to disaster (with special reference to Japan) [Powerpoint slides]. Retrieved from consultancy meeting "Global Radiation Medicine: Educational Challenges for Academia"

Clancey G (2013) Report to IAEA for technical meeting "Radiation, Health, and Society: Post-Fukushima Implications for the Training of Health Professionals". Vienna, 6–10 May

Danieli Y (ed) (1998) International handbook of multigenerational legacies of trauma. Plenum Press, New York

Fortun K, Frickel S (2012) Making a case for disaster science and technology studies: an STS Forum on Fukushima [Online forum]. http://fukushimaforum.wordpress.com/online-forum-2/online-forum/making-a-case-for-disaster-science-and-technology-studies/. Accessed 20 June 2013

Hamblin JD (2012) Fukushima and the motifs of nuclear history. Environ Hist 17(2):285–299. doi:10.1093/envhis/ems001

Hasegawa A, Miyazaki M, Tase C, Kumagai A, Ohtsuru A (2012) Fukushima Daiichi nuclear power plant accident and emergency medical response at Fukushima Medical University Hospital. In: The 6th international symposium of Nagasaki University Global COE Program "Global Strategic Center for Radiation Health Risk Control": a new challenge of radiation health risk management, Nagasaki, 20–22 Oct 2011, Nagasaki Publication, Showado, pp. 175–180

Hayashi K, Tomita N (2012) Lessons learned from the Great East Japan earthquake: impact on child and adolescent health. Asia Pac J Public Health 24(4):681–688. doi:10.1177/1010539512453255

International Atomic Energy Agency (1957) The statute of the International Atomic Energy Agency, art. II. http://www.iaea.org/About/statute.html. Accessed 23 July 2013

Kamiya K, Okamoto T, Hosoi Y (2012) Challenges and opportunities for strengthening global radiation medicine education: experiences of Hiroshima University [Powerpoint slides]. Retrieved from consultancy meeting "Global Radiation Medicine: Educational Challenges for Academia"

Matsuda N (2012) Six days in Fukushima: initial activities as a member of radiation emergency medical assistance team from Nagasaki. In: The 6th international symposium of Nagasaki University Global COE Program "Global Strategic Center for Radiation Health Risk Control": a new challenge of radiation health risk management, Nagasaki, 20–22 Oct 2011, Nagasaki Publication, Showado, pp 193–196

NIRS (2012) Reference document on education and self-study related to radiation medicine in medical education. http://www.nirs.go.jp/publication/igaku_siryo/igaku_siryo_e.pdf. Accessed 23 July 2013

NPR Staff and Wires (2011) Millions of stricken Japanese lack water, food, heat. NPR. http://www.npr.org/2011/03/18/134527591/millions-of-stricken-japanese-lack-water-food-heat. Accessed 20 June 2013

Nuclear and Industrial Safety Agency (2011) Regarding the evaluation of the conditions on reactor cores of unit 1, 2 and 3 related to the accident at Fukushima Daiichi Nuclear Power Station. Tokyo Electric Power Co. Inc. [Press release]. http://www.nsr.go.jp/archive/nisa/english/press/2011/06/en20110615-5.pdf. Accessed 20 June 2013

Okamoto T, Kamiya K, Hosoi Y (2012) Phoenix leader education program (Hiroshima Initiative) for renaissance from radiation disaster [Powerpoint slides]. Retrieved from consultancy meeting "Global Radiation Medicine: Educational Challenges for Academia"

Ozawa H, Dayuan N, Kusumoto Y, Kinoshita H, Imamura A (2011) Disaster psychiatry on earthquake and nuclear crisis in Fukushima. In: The 6th international symposium of Nagasaki University Global COE Program "Global Strategic Center for Radiation Health Risk Control": a new challenge of radiation health risk management, Nagasaki, 20–22 Oct 2011, Nagasaki Publication, Showado, p 93

Palgi Y, Ban-Ezra M, Aviel O, Dubiner Y, Baruch E, Soffer Y, Shrira A (2012) Mental health and disaster related attitudes among Japanese after the 2011 Fukushima nuclear disaster. J Psychiatr Res 46(5):688–690. doi:10.1016/j.jpsychires.2012.01.028

Practical Arrangements between the International Atomic Energy Agency and Fukushima Medical University (2012) Cooperation in the area of human health. 14 Dec 2012

Sakai K (2011) Issues on radiation exposure in the Fukushima nuclear accident – health effects, radiation protection, and public communication. In: The 6th international symposium of Nagasaki University Global COE Program "Global Strategic Center for Radiation Health Risk Control": a new challenge of radiation health risk management, Nagasaki, 20–22 Oct 2011, Nagasaki Publication, Showado, p 17

Takamura N (2012) Nagasaki University approaches to global radiation health challenges and practices [Powerpoint slides]. Retrieved from consultancy meeting "Global Radiation Medicine: Educational Challenges for Academia"

The Economist (2011) A crisis of leadership, too. The Economist Newspaper Ltd. http://www.economist.com/node/18441143. Accessed 10 June 2013

Wheeler B, Dotson S (2011) Japan's nuclear crisis: timeline of events. Power Eng 115(6):60–64

Yamashita S, Kumagai A (2012a) Fukushima Medical University approaches to global radiation health challenges and practices [Powerpoint slides]. Retrieved from consultancy meeting "Global Radiation Medicine: Educational Challenges for Academia"

Yamashita S, Kumagai A (2012b) Fukushima disaster medical seminars [Powerpoint slides]. Retrieved from consultancy meeting "Global Radiation Medicine: Educational Challenges For Academia"

Index

A

Acute radiation syndrome (ARS)
  characteristics, 69
  clinical symptoms
    dose and dose-rates, 70
    granulocyte and lymphocyte levels, 70
    nausea, vomiting and diarrhea, 70
    planning, 70
    and prognosis, 70
  description, 68
  high-dose injuries, 69
  symptoms, 22
  treatments
    and HS, 71, 72
    multi organ dysfunction syndrome, 71–72
ALARA. *See* As Low As Reasonably Achievable (ALARA)
Ambiguous losses
  Fukushima evacuees, 85
  government restrictions, 85
  radioactive contamination, tsunami, 84
  suicidal cases, 85
ARS. *See* Acute radiation syndrome (ARS)
As Low As Reasonably Achievable (ALARA), 25

B

Biological effects, radiation disaster medicine
  acute effects, 22
  deterministic effects, 21, 22
  gastrointestinal symptoms, 22
  human, 22
  ICRP, 22–23
  living cells, 21
  stochastic effects, 22

C

CBRNE. *See* Chemical, biological, radiological, nuclear and explosives (CBRNE) events
CDPC. *See* Central Disaster Prevention Council (CDPC)
Central Disaster Prevention Council (CDPC), 92
Chemical, biological, radiological, nuclear and explosives (CBRNE) events, 58
Chronic anxiety and guilt, 84
Clancey, G., 112
Corrigan, P.W., 86

D

Decontamination, hospital emergency medical response
  life-saving measurement, 66
  MCE, 66
  partial body, 66, 67
  REA, 66
  skin/wound damage, 66
  worker with head contamination, 66
Deterministic effects, radiation, 21, 22
Disaster behavioral health. *See* Fukushima Daiichi Nuclear Power Plant Accident
Disaster Medical Assistance Teams (DMATs)
  inpatient evacuations, 31, 32
  in Japan, 55, 56
  Ministry of Health, labor and welfare, 51
Disaster related death (DRD), 45
DMATs. *See* Disaster Medical Assistance Teams (DMATs)
Dose assessment, 67, 68
DRD. *See* Disaster related death (DRD)

K. Tanigawa, R.K. Chhem (eds.), *Radiation Disaster Medicine*,
DOI 10.1007/978-3-319-02216-1, © Springer International Publishing Switzerland 2014

E

Emergency physicians, 6

F

Family and community physicians
- emergency situation, 7
- hospital facilities, 6–7
- laboratory/X-ray tests, 7

Fukushima accident
- anxious hospital staff, 73, 75
- chronology, events, 46, 47
- Daiichi NPP, 51, 52
- DMAT, 51
- 5/6 ER, 51–54
- evacuated patients, 50
- experiences from, 34
- Great East Japan Earthquake, 55–57
- hospital staff and medical assistant teams, 73, 74
- hypothermia, 51
- injuries and illnesses, 46, 48–49
- medical facility, J-Village, 51, 52
- NPP and FMU, 72, 73
- radiation emergency medical system, 46, 47, 72
- road conditions, 53
- TEPCO Fukushima Nuclear Power Plant Emergency Medical System Network, 53, 55
- time reduction, radiation exposure, 34–35

Fukushima Daiichi Nuclear Power Plant Accident
- behavioral effects, nuclear accidents (*see* Nuclear disasters)
- behavioral health problems, 80
- "Hama-Dori", 80
- high-risk groups, 87
- nuclear fallouts, 80
- physicians' early response (*see* Physicians' early response)
- psychological consequences
  - ambiguous losses, 84–85
  - chronic anxiety and guilt, 84
  - features of, people after accident, 82, 83
  - posttraumatic stress responses, 82–84
  - separated families and communities, 85–86
  - stigma and self-stigma, 86
- radioactive substances, ^{134}Cs and ^{137}Cs, 80
- risk communication and programs, 87

Fukushima Medical University (FMU)
- decontamination facilities, 59, 66
- radiation accidents, 73
- and REA, 62, 63, 65

G

Geriatricians, 7

Great East Japan Earthquake
- DMATs, 56
- JAAM, 55–57
- JATEC, 55
- medical care, disasters, 55

H

Hematologists and transfusion medicine physicians, 7–8

Hematopoietic syndrome (HS), 71, 72

Hospital emergency medical response
- ARS (*see* Acute radiation syndrome (ARS))
- decontamination, 66, 67
- description, 58
- dose assessment, 67, 68
- Fukushima accident, 72–75
- IAEA, 60–61
- LRI, 68, 69
- MCEs, 60, 64
- patient reception, 64, 65
- planning, 58–59
- preparation
  - medical staff, 63–64
  - patients' arrival, 61, 62
  - REA, 61–63
  - survey meters, 64
- radiological evaluation (*see* Radiological evaluation)
- triage and life-saving treatment, 64
- workers injured clinical data, hydrogen explosion, 60

HS. *See* Hematopoietic syndrome (HS)

I

IAEA. *See* International Atomic Energy Agency (IAEA)

ICRP. *See* International Commission on Radiological Protection (ICRP)

IEC. *See* Incident and Emergency Centre (IEC)

IEComm. *See* Incident and Emergency Communication (IEComm)

Incident and Emergency Centre (IEC)
  of IAEA, 101
  on-call officers, 101
Incident and Emergency Communication (IEComm), 105–106
Injury Severity Score (ISS), 42
International Atomic Energy Agency (IAEA), 60–61
  Chernobyl disaster, 81
  conventions
    assistance, nuclear accident/radiological emergency, 101
    early notification, nuclear accident, 100
  and TMI, 81
International Commission on Radiological Protection (ICRP), 22, 34
International organizations (IO)
  contact personnel, radiation disasters, 106–107
  conventions, IAEA (*see* International Atomic Energy Agency (IAEA))
  description, 100
  and IEC (*see* Incident and Emergency Centre (IEC))
  IEComm, 105–106
  Joint Plan, 101–104
  JPLAN, 105
  protocols and operational arrangements, 105
  RANET, 106
  technical documents and websites, 100
IO. *See* International organizations (IO)
ISS. *See* Injury Severity Score (ISS)

J

JAAM. *See* Japan Association for Acute Medicine (JAAM)
Japan Association for Acute Medicine (JAAM)
  Fukushima, 56
  and JAST, 55
  and JSDF, 57
Japanese Advanced Trauma Evaluation and Care (JATEC), 55
Japan, radiation emergency response
  countermeasures, nuclear disasters, 92
  disaster medicine, 90
  education, training and exercise/drills, 95–96
  history of
    accidents and incidents, 90, 91
    CDPC, 92
    NIRS, 92
    TEPCO Fukushima Daiichi NPP, 92
  medical response, 90
  public concerns, 96–97
  radiation accident, 90
  response system (*see* Response system)
  symptoms/signs, 90
  temporary house-visit program, 96
Japan Self Defense Forces (JSDF), 59, 95
JATEC. *See* Japanese Advanced Trauma Evaluation and Care (JATEC)
Joint Radiation Emergency Management Plan (JPLAN), 105
JPLAN. *See* Joint Radiation Emergency Management Plan (JPLAN)
JSDF. *See* Japan Self Defense Forces (JSDF)
J-Village
  command center, nuclear accident, 40
  description, 40
  Fukushima Daiichi NPP, 51
  JFA National Training Center, 41
  medical facility in, 52

K

Kasl, S.V., 81
Kereiakes, J.G., 5
Kyutoku, Y., 83

L

LET. *See* Linear energy transfer (LET)
Level of consciousness (LOC), 40
Linear energy transfer (LET), 19
LOC. *See* Level of consciousness (LOC)
Local radiation injury (LRI)
  clinical symptoms, 68, 69
  description, 68
  ulceration and necrosis, 68
LRI. *See* Local radiation injury (LRI)

M

Mass casualty event (MCE)
  component, emergency response system, 31
  DMATs, 31, 32
  evacuation planning, 31
  explosion, 17
  field care and patient triage, 31
  medical teams, 31
  PPE and radiation meters, 31

Mass casualty event (MCE) (*cont.*)
  protocols, 31
  radiation disaster, 31
  regional and national resources, 31–32
MCE. *See* Mass casualty event (MCE)
Medical perspective
  hospital emergency medical response (*see* Hospital emergency medical response)
  pre-hospital emergency medical response (*see* Pre-hospital emergency medical response)

N
Nephrologists, 8
Nuclear disasters
  Chernobyl disaster, 81
  cleanup workers, 81
  cognitive functioning, exposed infants, 81–82
  Japanese psychiatrists, 82
  JCO, 82
  non-supervisory workers, TMI, 81
  posttraumatic stress disorder, 82
  psychological impacts, 80–81
  temporal profile groups, 81
  TMI and IAEA, 81
Nuclear medicine physicians, 5

O
Occupational health physicians (TEPCO workers), 9
Orthopedic surgeons and anesthetists, 8

P
Pediatricians, 8–9
Personal protective equipment (PPE)
  in-house triage area, 39
  and radiation meters, 31
  radioactive materials, 33, 34
Physicians' early response
  CanMeds physician competency framework, 2, 3
  communicators, 10–11
  description, 2
  emergency physicians, 6
  family and community physicians, 6–7
  geriatricians, 7
  hematologists and transfusion medicine physicians, 7–8
  nephrologists, 8
  nuclear medicine physicians, 5
  occupational health physicians (TEPCO workers), 9
  orthopedic surgeons and anesthetists, 8
  pediatricians, 8–9
  professionals, 9–10
  psychiatrists, 9
  pulmonary specialists, 8
  radiation disaster medicine, 4–5
  radiologists, 5
  radio-oncologists, 6
  RCPSC 2009, 2, 4
Post-Fukushima context
  approach, STS (*see* Science and Technology Studies (STS))
  authorities and experts, 111
  "crisis in expertise", 111
  disaster medical seminars, 114–115
  earthquake, tsunami and nuclear accident, 110
  FMU, 114
  Hiroshima University, 114
  hydrogen explosions, 110
  IAEA, 111
  internet and social media, 111
  Japan Standard Time (JST), 110
  lack, nuclear emergency preparedness, 111
  Nagasaki University, 114
  NAHU/IAEA, 112–113
  NIRS, 115
  Project NA9/16, 115–116
  Project NA9/17, 116–117
Posttraumatic stress responses
  earthquakes and tsunami, 82
  explosion at plant, 84
  hyperarousal and reexperiencing symptoms, 83
  meltdown and radioactive exposure, 83
  psychiatric clinics, Fukushima Prefecture, 83
PPE. *See* Personal protective equipment (PPE)
Pre-hospital emergency medical response
  characterized, radiation disaster, 30
  command center, 40–41
  Fukushima accident (*see* Fukushima accident)
  public health consequences, 44–46
  on radiation
    dose rate/prediction, spread pattern, 41
    mobile monitoring posts, 41
    portable monitoring posts, 41–42

public safety, 41
SPEEDI, 41
re-establishment (*see* Re-establishment, medical response system)
workers, 42–44
Primary ABCDE approach
medical evaluation, 64
patients with life-threatening conditions, 40
Prince-Embury, S., 81
Psychiatrists, 9
Public health consequences
disaster related death (DRD), 45
Fukushima accident, 45
Great East Japan earthquake, 45
life conditions, 44
medical activities, Tohoku regions, 45
officials and organization, 45–46
restricted zone, 44

R

Radiation disaster medicine
accidents, 16
ALARA, 25
alpha and beta particles, 18
biological effects (*see* Biological effects, radiation disaster medicine)
catastrophic natural events, 16
description, 16
experts in, 4–5
external exposure and contamination
Chernobyl accident, 20–21
description, 20
Fukushima accident, 21
legal radiation exposure, 20
flow of energy, 18
gamma rays, 18
humans and animals, 18
initial evaluation, victim, 24
LET, 19
levels, care, 17
magnitude, 16–17
MCE, 17
medical needs, 17
natural/man-made, 16
neutrons, 19
personnel and objectives, 17
principle, emergency medical approaches, 26
radioactive dusts and plume, 23
radioactive iodine-131 (^{131}I) and radioactive cesium-137 (^{137}Cs), 18
radionuclides and radiations, 18, 19
sophisticated radiological survey systems, 17
survey meters, 24–25
trauma, 23, 24
ultraviolet light and waves of mobile phones, 18
Radiation emergency area (REA)
decontamination and treatment rooms, 61
main traffic flow, 61
non-contaminated patients, 61
outside entrance/easy access, 61
and patient reception, 64, 65
preparation, 61, 63
ventilation, 61
Radiation emergency response
IO (*see* International organizations (IO))
in Japan (*see* Japan, radiation emergency response)
"Radiation-society interaction" conceptual framework, 112
Radiological evaluation
decontamination, 66
done prior, 64
nasal swabs, 64
survey meter, 65
and treatment, 64, 65
victim's condition, 65
Radiologists, 5
Radio-oncologists, 6
RANET. *See* Response and Assistance Network (RANET)
Raphael, B., 84
REA. *See* Radiation emergency area (REA)
Re-establishment, medical response system
ambient radiation, 34
emergency personnel, 33
Fukushima accident, 34–35
huge earthquake, 31
ICRP, 34
initial information, 33
management, on-site response in radiation disaster
austere environment, 37
explosion, 36
in-house triage and treatment area, 36
medical team, 36
PPE, 35–36
restricted area, 35
safety zone, 35
MCE and inpatient evacuation, 31–32
nuclear reactor accident, 34
Persian blue (PB), 34

Re-establishment, medical response system (*cont.*)
potassium iodide (KI), 34
PPE, 33
radiation accidents, 33, 34
radioactive materials, 33, 34
treatment
airway problems, 40
austere circumstances, 40
breathing, 40
chest trauma, 40
LOC, 40
PPE in-house triage area, 39
primary ABCDE approach, 40
triage and on-site decontamination
absorption, radioactive materials, 39
categories, radiation injuries, 37, 38
clinical symptoms, 37
external contamination, 38
pre-hospital triage, radiation disaster, 37
START, 37
treatment priority, 37
water, 39
wet decontamination, 38
Response and Assistance Network (RANET), 106
Response system
cytogenetic and physical dose assessments, 95
JSDF, 95
NIRS, 93
patients accidentally exposed and/or contaminated, 93, 94
prefectures, nuclear facilities (NFs), 93
rescues, helicopters, 95
three levels, radiation emergency hospitals, 93, 94
UPZ of NPPs, 95
Rooney, J.F., 81

S
Science and Technology Studies (STS)
components, NAHU, 114
"radiation-society interaction" problems, 113
residents, Japan, 113
scientific and technical expertise, 113
techno scientific disasters, 113
Separated families and communities
epidemiological study, 85
members and evacuees, 86
multiple factors, 85
natural disasters, 85
types of discordance, 85–86
Shigemura, J., 86
Simple triage and rapid treatment (START), 37
START. *See* Simple triage and rapid treatment (START)
Stigma and self-stigma, 86
STS. *See* Science and Technology Studies (STS)

T
Temporary house-visit program, 96
TEPCO Fukushima Nuclear Power Plant Emergency Medical System Network, 53, 55
"The Chromosome Analysis Network Council", 95
"The Physical Dosimetry Network Council", 95
Three Mile Island (TMI)
and IAEA, 81
non-supervisory workers, 81
workers of, 81
TMI. *See* Three Mile Island (TMI)

U
UPZ. *See* Urgent Protective Action Planning Zone (UPZ)
Urgent Protective Action Planning Zone (UPZ), 95

W
Workers, pre-hospital emergency medical response
acute myocardial infarction, 42
general fatigue and sickness, 42
heat stroke, 42
injuries and illnesses, 42, 43
irradiation dose
disaster stricken areas, 44, 45
nuclear reactor accident, 44
TEPCO, 43
total radiation dose, 42–43
ISS, 42
restoration operations, accident facility, 42

MIX
Papier aus verantwortungsvollen Quellen
Paper from responsible sources
FSC® C105338

If you have any concerns about our products,
you can contact us on
ProductSafety@springernature.com

In case Publisher is established outside the EU,
the EU authorized representative is:
Springer Nature Customer Service Center GmbH
Europaplatz 3, 69115 Heidelberg, Germany

Printed by Libri Plureos GmbH
in Hamburg, Germany